A Life on Pause

Brianna D. Harris-Henderson

Table of Contents

Chapter 1   An Almost Perfect Life

Chapter 2   Through Sickness & In Health

Chapter 3   A Turn for The Worst

Chapter 4   Waiting to Prevail

Chapter 5   An Unconditional Healing

Chapter 6   A Beautiful Nightmare

Chapter 7   I'm Broken to Heal

Chapter 8   Every Reason to Praise God

Chapter 9   A Life on Pause

Dedication

This book is dedicated to those who have been broken many times but refuse to give up on themselves. The patient with a rare or common disease who no one seems to understand. The complicated teenage girl who's lost a mother at a young age. Those who may feel alone even while sitting in a room filled with hundreds of people.

I thank my Lord and Savior, as it was he who put this book on my heart while being patient with me as he allowed my tears to speak healing to my heart, my amazing children for being the best they can be, my dear husband for always being by my side, and lovely immediate family for always supporting my quirky ideas.

Inspired by my own hopes, and dreams."

About the Book

Feeling trapped in a world of grief, love, financial, and heath struggles, Brianna grew up feeling that her life's purpose did not exist. As she remains resiliant through all the traumatic emotional events, she finds herself becoming a CEO, patients advocate, public speaker, doula, grant writer, and published author. With all thanks to God, she believes he prepared her for the worst to only bring out her best, to help heal others around the nation.

CHAPTER 1

An Almost Perfect Life

I tell many people that my illness was not a punishment but an assignment in my life led by God. You see, he spared my life twice amid the enemy trying to destroy me. Once after, I experienced a severe postpartum hemorrhage, and second, being diagnosed with stage three heart failure at the age of 23. At first, it was hard to believe that God had placed a calling on my life because I wasn't always a loving and caring person. I was not a very good friend to others and didn't do well staying connected with my family.

Once I gained knowledge from the Bible in my teen years, God opened my eyes to the person I would soon become. But because I didn't believe it, it took a while longer to guide me there. Along the way, he set some trials and tribulations in place to move me in the direction of bringing others, young or old, back to him. His spiritual guidance taught me to discern quickly, to hear his voice, and not to cast judgment. It taught me to develop a strategy to help broken people find their way back to God. The healing is in our Lord and Savior, and to receive that, we must be willing to read and understand his Basic Information Before Leaving Earth (Bible).

As a child, I was vulnerable to the real world before realizing it would soon be against me. Being the tenth child on my dad's side and the second for my mother made it no better. Yet, I felt there was something unique about me that others couldn't see. I was born and raised in Texas in a lovely home with my big sister Crystal, my mother Precious, and my dad Ricci. My sister and I were seven years apart, but we bonded in the best way God allowed us to. I once read that "having a sister is probably the biggest love/hate relationship you'll ever experience. Still, sisters have a bond like no other, whether you're the responsible big sister or the wild child little sister; you know what you have is special, especially a sister of the same womb." That was the exact type of bond my sister and I had over the years, and no matter what happened, we had one another.

I was unaware that God could choose anyone he wants to do his will or fulfill a purpose in life until I read some biblical stories related to my life one day. Looking back over the years, I never thought I'd become a motivational speaker, spiritual influencer, patient advocate, businesswoman, or founder of an organization led by strong, inspiring, resilient women. To think of it, I never even knew I was special in God's eyes because of the distractions the enemy had been blinding me with most of my life. I always loved making people laugh, smile, or uplift their spirits in any way I could. Yet, in return, I'd be the one to be taken advantage of, stabbed in the back, or be highly misunderstood. At a young age, I taught myself that humans are like turtles, cruising slowly in life, waiting for God to pick them up and place them where they want to be. Turtles all have shells, so we cannot see what's on the inside until it's removed. As a human turtle, you aren't aware of what's under another person's shell until God reveals and removes them.

By the time I was born, my dad had become a filmaholic creating daily mini-movies when we were living in these small two-bedroom apartments in Pleasant Grove. A little after turning one, my mom had been looking for us a three-bed home, and with her and my dad's income, they were approved. Our parents always came up with many fun activities during our childhood, traveling, vacations, and tons of other special memories we enjoyed. Our parents did a wonderful job raising us. There was never a sorrowful moment under our roof, but life was never perfect.

I was the ringleader in daycare, teaching other babies how to crawl out of the playpen and be free. At home, I would pretend I was a ballerina and prance around the house in my favorite tutu after attending my sister's dance competitions. When I was five, I begged my parents to put me on "Barney." I loved the show, but our names would never get selected for auditioning. Mom even worked with a woman who had her son on it, but it didn't get us in.

My mom worked for the FDA, so somedays I would tag along with her to shadow all she did. She was very talented in her position and brilliant at how she handled business. I was four going on five when I started school, thanks to my parents for making me a valentine's baby. On my first day of school, no one mentioned how exhausting and difficult it would be to get up out of bed early. As the day went on, we went from introductions to hand painting. I even had the chance to see my sister Crystal during lunchtime. She walked over to my classmates and I to hand me a giant chocolate chip cookie that she bought. All my classmates were like, "ahh, who is that girl?" and I was proud to say, "oh, that's my big sister!" It was her last year in elementary school, so it felt good having that experience being there together. We were the complete opposite of each other. She was the sweet, discreet, and upstanding one. I, on the other hand, was the sour, surreptitious, and intrepid one, but we understood one another.

For my 7th birthday, momma booked a clown to entertain the family and me at home for my party. I felt like a magical princess that day, and the clown made me feel even more like it when she had me do a fun magic trick in front of our guests. "I MADE CANDY APPEAR!" I shouted those words, and we ate it all night.

Just about every night, when getting ready for bed, our mom or dad would come into our room and make sure we read a page from the children's Bible that included a nightly prayer. We weren't an 'every Sunday' church-going family, but the days we attended, I couldn't understand the importance of listening to the pastor.

One night, I awoke from a nightmare that my mom and sister both died in a car accident. I quickly rushed into my parent's room to check my mom's breathing and went across the hall to check on Crystal's breathing. They were both fine, so I was confused about why I would have a dream like that. I never told them about it, but I knew to cherish them daily. In 2001 Crystal became captain of her school's drill team and brought home shiny gold trophies that I unknowingly admired.

One afternoon, we had an event program where I saw the school's drill team perform. I had seemed to be the only one in my class interested, so I asked my mom privately to find out about the team. She was told that I had to wait until I was in 3rd grade to try out. In the meantime, I was placed in a talented and gifted program after my parents were told I was a very bright child.

In 2002 I became a 3rd grader and couldn't wait to join the school's dance team. I had never been so determined before in my whole nine years of life. On meet the teacher night, momma and I met the lady who would be my teacher and was also the coach for the drill team! She gave us the try-out information, and when that day came, I nailed it, giving it my all with a smile and attitude. Later that week, I found out I made the team and was too proud of myself.

Dancing was like being a superstar, but without the famous

part. I finally knew what my sister felt like every time she would hit that stage. Anytime my performances would come up, mom had Crystal do my hair and critique me when I'd practice at home. We were a traveling family already, so when it came time to go on the road for competitions, my dad and I were all for it. He would go on a few trips with us through the year as a chaperone and van driver while mom and Crystal stayed home. Dance was my new life, and I loved every bit of it. That is until I started having a crush on one of my dance partners' brothers. I slowly became ashamed and developed a lack of confidence at each performance in front of him because mom didn't believe in shaving under a young girl's arms. So embarrassing, right? I was already given the name hairy Harris because of my hairy arms and legs that I hated so much. It wasn't until she had no choice but to get me shaved after our coach requested to have it done for all the dancers.

After going to school on a bad day, I got into my first fight with a classmate during recess. No adults saw us pushing each other, but all our classmates did and surrounded us to watch. Once school was out, I went to dancing practice as if nothing happened. I always tried not to let negative situations get to me because I'm normally a peacemaker or problem solver for others. When I started to dance, one of the main things we were told was to keep our grades up. The problem with that was I wasn't a good test taker, so it caused major roller coaster rides in my grades. Being a Pantherette at W.A. Blair kept me entertained with limited things to do in my free time and my focus off the stressors of school.

On some weekends, our other (half) siblings would come and stay with us. We enjoyed having another sister and three brothers around, but they eventually stopped coming as they got older. My brothers taught me how to play video games, and I became addicted. I was a complete game freak. As time went on, things started to get a little gloomy in the house. My sister and I were taught to mind our business, so we didn't focus much on the lives our parents were living that we weren't aware of. We would attend family reunions every year on both sides, but my dad's side always picked places to travel to versus mom's side that went to the same spot since it's in Fairfield, Tx.

One strange day, Crystal shared an uncanny story with me that one of our cousins, who was in 10th grade at the time, told the family. Our cousin noticed a student in her class one evening who she thought looked like our dad, so she randomly asked the girl who her dad was. The girl said she wasn't sure, but she'd ask her mother to find out. The next day, the girl returned with a name, and it was indeed our dad! We were all stunned at the news, but he explained and cleared things up to give us some type of understanding.

Although there was nothing that could be done, our mom didn't take the information too kindly it was a complete shock to her. It caused some rockiness in their marriage, and only the worse was about to come. I thought it was pretty cool that I had more siblings and wanted to meet and spend time with them. The following year, dad planned a mini trip with a rent-a-van for all 11 of his kids; to have a sleepover while getting to know one another. It wasn't something that normally happened in life, but it did in ours. In between the months that were passing, I'd go to school and pretend nothing drastic was going on at home, and by the summertime, dad planned a family cruise for just us, my grandma (paternal), and cousin. Mom let us know that she was not going to be a part of the trip, so I was sort of disappointed that she wasn't, but I tried to understand her why.

Carnival cruise was my first time being on a huge boat, and the room dad picked out was so nice! We traveled to Cozumel, Calica, and The Grand Cayman Islands in five days. We called momma each time we docked to check on her and express how much we wished she was there. Everything was so beautiful. The view of the dolphins following our boat, the swish sounds of the ocean, and how pretty the bluish water was. I knew then this would be something I'd be into when I grew up. Crystal and I had a great time and couldn't wait to get back home to show mom pictures. After making it home and getting settled, something had been on momma's mind, but she had no way to release it.

A few weeks passed, and she slowly grew lack of interest in going to work. She went to her PCP and was diagnosed with "major depressive disorder." Whatever it was that bothered her became worse in a short amount of time. She was such a wonderful woman, literally. One night my granny(maternal) mentioned to her about an uncle that was struggling with food. We all went with her to the grocery store and were attacked by dog fleas while walking to their door to deliver the groceries. She would even plan out the family activities for our yearly family reunions and was just the life of the party. She was hardworking, determined, compassionate, humorous, kind-hearted, and a generous person as long as no one pushed her buttons, or she'd be ready to set things straight!

Apparently, mom continued feeling sentimental and decided that separation or divorce from dad would best. I couldn't believe our joyful household was falling apart like this. I did my best to ignore what was going on and stay focused in school to keep my grades up for dance. The pain eventually started to weigh down on me, becoming more of a distraction since I had always been a daddy's girl. It was so heartbreaking watching them go through this, and after a few monotonous months, dad found a nice townhome not too far from home. I finally understood what those kids who dealt with separated parents felt like, especially going back and forth between houses. Dad meant well in all he did and was very dedicated to taking care of his family in every way a man should. I grew up watching him do some of the most important and coolest things I didn't see in other homes.

CHAPTER TWO

Through Sickness & In Health

Between 2002 and 2004, I was slowly adapting to the new normal life that snuck into our lives. Both of my parents were doing well on their own until one night, dad had this weird dream about God instructing him to return home. He didn't understand the dream but received confirmation from my grandma to obey the message. A few days later, he made a phone call explaining to mom that he needed to move back home. She was stunned, but allowed him to come back, making it clear that they would not be in the same room. She had just begun feeling like a new woman, living life to the fullest, traveling, and making us happy the best she could. One night mom was gone for a while, but when she returned, there was the cutest puppy in her hands that she bought for me since Crystal wasn't a big fan of animals. We had always been a dog family, and after the tragic loss of our original family dog, Fluffy filled the emptiness in our hearts.

When she announced that dad was moving back home, I was too excited and felt things were finally coming together after two long years of separation. He moved back in but stayed in the guest area part of the house to give them both continued space. About two months later, my sister and I found out that mom and granny were not on the best of terms after mom came out with a painful secret she's held in for many years. Mom made us aware that the man we've known as our nonbiological grandpa molested her when she was only a pre-teen. This had explained to us why mom was so big when it came to certain men in our life or any man for that matter. She trained our minds well, but we never knew what happened to her. Our granny had a hard time believing it at first, but after a day or two, she moved away after a confrontation with him. I felt bad for my granny because that's the man she's spent the majority of her life with.

Due to this unexpected situation, granny came to live with us until she was able to find a new place to stay. Unfortunately, she had to share a room with me, but I was totally fine with that since I used to spend the night with her all the time. Overall, it was an overwhelming feeling of joy having all of us under one roof and attending all my dance performances. The energy in the house was very different, and a few weeks later, I found out why. One evening, when mom came home, she had been feeling this pea-size knot in her breast and asked dad to inspect it. He told her to make an appointment to rule out anything serious, and within a week, it had grown a quarter in size. During her appointment, the doctor did a biopsy on her breast. A biopsy is a way an oncologist evaluates a suspicious area in the breast to determine whether it is cancerous.

That late evening, granny called me in the room, saying mom was on the phone and wanted to talk to me. She stated she was on her way home but found out some bad news. She said, "The doctor said momma had cancer in the breast, but we're going to pray about it and get through this." I said, "Oh no, momma!" while shedding a few tears. I was 10 years old, so I was in the dark about how serious things could be. The following week the knot grew into a golf ball size, then a few days later, it was baseball size. A mastectomy surgery was strongly recommended, and as our mother's number one supporters, we discussed every option as a family. She went ahead and got the breast removal done, and soon afterwards the oncologist came out to update everyone.

He explained to my dad that mom's lymph nodes were destroyed by cancer, but they removed all the cancer cells that could be seen. After going through so much in such a short time, mom remained strong and resilient. The side effects from the chemo and radiation made all of her hair fall out, along with burning skin to where it would peel and bleed.

After a few months, it was time for her to undergo a tummy tuck procedure to rebuild a breast and nipple to replace the old one. At this point, my grades started slipping, and I slowly was ready to give up. The time I spent at school was more time away from her. One evening momma gained enough energy and took me to my 4th-grade parent-teacher conference. She brought pictures of what she had gone through in hopes that my teacher would understand why my focus was not all there. Unfortunately, most schools don't care about what a child is going through at home unless they're being abused in some way. Only three teachers cared.

Mom became a breast cancer survivor at the end of 2004, and to celebrate with her, we joined a 'Race for the Cure' walk. She felt blessed to be there and was thankful to have a second chance at life. Mom and dad even made up, started working on their relationship, and she returned to work. While things were going great at home, I was hit with the news that my coach was ending the dance team due to her becoming a new mother. It was a very devastating moment because I was going to miss the eyelashes, long genie ponytails, the body glitter, and how it felt to perform on stage. On the plus side, I was glad to have been co-captain for our last year. During the mix of things, granny was able to get back on her feet and move into her new place and Crystal was surprised with a new car for her birthday.

One school morning, momma woke up with a severe headache and couldn't drop me off, so Crystal did. The following week she tried to take fluffy to the groomers but couldn't properly drive with a constant headache. When I was a baby, my dad lost his oldest sister to a brain tumor, and mom remembered some symptoms. She asked dad to refresh her memory on it, and as he explained everything, he said we weren't claiming that. She made an appointment the following week, and mom prepared herself for whatever the results would be. Her brain scans came in, which revealed a tumor was sitting directly in the middle of her brain. The oncologist confirmed that the cells from the breast cancer had traveled to a spot in the brain that they wouldn't be able to remove.

Our biological grandpa(maternal) had flown in from ATL to help us out around the house and spend time with mom. Once she started chemo and radiation again, my mother decided to let him shave all the new hair she had finally grown back. She was so brave, and strong so that's all we could see. The oncologist explained that there was nothing more they could do, and to prepare for her condition to get worse. However, he did start prescribing a lot of pain and sleeping medications which she began needing as the weeks passed. Nights would come where momma would just start screaming in agony because she could not rest in bed without pain. This lasted for at least a week until she found comfort laying on the sofa sleeper in the living room. To keep her company Crystal and I would watch T.V. or movies with her all day sometimes, or we'd just rest along with her.

Mommas' pain became more severe each night, so her doctor prescribed her some steroid medication to help with pain and energy. She had developed some strength and became very hyperactive when it came to helping others or spending money. One day my sister was upset with tears in her eyes because momma decided to give her car away, but she assured her she'd get another one. Later that week, mom took us to a car lot and bought Crystal a brand new car that was a lot better than the last one. Though she was getting more ill, she could still drive and do pretty much normal things that she had the interest to do.

One night we needed to go to the store, so she took us to target. She grabbed a basket and went down every single aisle, throwing items in it. Crystal kept telling her to put a lot of the things back, but mom had become a little more aggressive with her actions. We never thought we would get out of there, especially since daddy wasn't with us to help get her out of the store. This was not the first time she had done this, but this was the first time we were alone with her without help. She caused a dramatic scene in front of the store because Crystal called to tell dad what she was doing. He was working overtime, so he couldn't do anything but tell the manager that she was very ill and unaware of her behavior. They even called security on us, so embarrassing! After our grandpa traveled went back home, granny came back to stay a few nights to help dad get enough sleep for work. He had used all of his medical leave taking care of the house.

Chapter Three

A Turn for The Worst

I started leaving on weekends to go to my big cousin's house, just trying to find a new environment. My cousin's main thing was making sure we got up for church and ate a good breakfast every Sunday. It was always a great time being there, and on the plus side, I liked being a part of a diverse children's church with friendly kids. One night at home, mom was so energized that she walked around the whole house opening up windows and turning on every light in the house.

No matter how tough it got, I still had to attend school, and focus the best I could. Yet there was a serious mental struggle going on that no one understood. We had to get my mom medical attention one night because the medicine kept her awake. She was quickly given a room, but it took them a while to calm her down because she was putting on a show for their cameras, acting like she was Martin Lawrence when he played the security guard, Otis.

They decided to keep her overnight to give her a somnolent medication, so we could all try to get some decent sleep.

Mom would receive tons of visitors from co-workers to teachers, friends, and family. There were so many people that it was hard to keep up with them. Some days momma would lay in the bedroom and have a some family or old friends come to see her, so she didn't have to get up. Later that day, mom noticed her wedding ring was no longer on the dresser, and the only ones who had come in were family. She had a feeling about who took it, but she was not about to focus her energy on it. My sister and I sort of became used to having company, especially not having to worry about dinner some nights, because they always brought food or gifts. She did have a lot of caring and loving people there for her despite any enemies.

For my 12th birthday, mom planned a skating rink party with some of my classmates from school. She always knew exactly what to do to help take our minds off of things. We made it through Thanksgiving, but Christmas morning was different. I jumped up out of bed to wake up everyone, as I do every year in excitement.

Dad helped mom out of bed to watch us open gifts, and it was the first time I saw the tiredness in her eyes. That evening, we took her to a gathering dedicated to her that a family member put together; she enjoyed herself but was exhausted once leaving.

After we brought in the year 2006, dad had a meeting with mom's doctor about her struggling to walk. He told dad to start preparing all-important paperwork and to go ahead and medically retire her from work. He gave momma six months to live and that her health was going to decline rapidly. The next month she could no longer walk or even stand on her own two feet. She slowly stopped wanting certain meals and eventually only wanted smoothies. One of my great aunts had bought her a juicer, so I'd help dad slice up fruits and veggies to feed it to her. At this point, my dad needed major assistance, so hospice was brought in to provide 24hr health care. I loved meeting all the nurses who helped momma because they were always so sweet to us.

Dad and granny had to continue working, and Crystal was able to get a position at mommas job. Thank God for two grandmothers though, because my other grandma was able to come to sit with her some days through the week. They would talk about Biblical things together and sing gospel songs. Momma's favorite one was "Silver & Gold" by Kirk Franklin, following the scripture she quoted daily, "Psalms 23". God gifted my grandma in many amazing ways. She has been through the same process with her daughter she lost many years before. A few days later, momma no longer had an appetite and immediately started to lose a lot of weight.

I got home from school and ran to hug and speak to mom and told her I wanted to dance for her, so I did. She smiled at me, saying "Bri, you always have to be the center of attention." I laughed while continuing to prance around the room. At the end of that week, dad gathered Crystal and me to discuss plans on how things would go as mom's health grew worse. The next month, momma fell into a coma and needed to be placed on oxygen to help her breathe properly. We had one last gathering, and it was for everyone to sing happy early birthday to her because we weren't sure if she would still be there on May 14th.

April 24th came, and like any other day, I'd completed my normal scheduled routine that includes homework, eating dinner, a bath, saying prayers, and ready for bed. While I tried to get some sleep for school the next day, mommas feet begin turning purple, and her breathing became fainter. The hospice nurse went to wake up dad and suggest that he and Crystal get up and talk to her. A little after 1 am, mom took her last breath, and dad came to wake me up. I was so tired that I barely understood what was happening until he said, "Bri, momma was gone, she's with Jesus now". He walked me closer to her, but I was sort of frightened. He comforted me and said this was only the shell she lived in and that the spirit who made her momma was in heaven. Then I saw Crystal crying, leaning over the couch calling granny, but she waited to tell her the bad news.

The nurse took my hand to walk me up to momma, and I stood there with her until granny came through the door in tears. We comforted one another as we waited for the medical team to come time her death and wait for Lincoln Memorial funeral home to pick her up.

Fluffy had been staying next to her hospice bed since day one, and there he was on the corner, protecting her. Granny and I noticed how momma looked so peaceful, almost as if she were still sleeping. Her eyes were closed, but her teeth were showing like she passed away with a smile. She'll never know how it taught me to smile through anything because that's what she did. After the funeral home arrived, that whole moment became an interval. They entered the house with a stretcher, went into the room with mom, and closed us off. They had placed her in a black body bag and rolled her out on the stretcher while we all were pouring our hearts out. I saw the nurse packing up her things and kindly walked her to the door, thanking her for taking care of our mom. It warmed her heart, and as she left, she said, "Such a sweet-sweet girl Jesus." I quickly pulled myself together to make sure everyone else was okay because that was the most painful experience ever!

I went to sit on granny's lap at the kitchen table, and we both glanced in the room mom was in, looking in the now-empty bed. Dad called my school to let everyone know that I would be out the rest of the week, so they made a special announcement for me. The next morning some hospice workers came to get their equipment, and I quickly snatched off mom's cushion pillow. I missed her so much already but had no clue how to express it without having her here to hug on. Throughout her last days, it was difficult hugging or loving on her, because of the pain her body would be in. I cried in my room, asking God to help with the pain I felt because I didn't know what to do. I started texting a few of my friends, but all they could say was "sorry for your loss" or "oh my gosh, I heard what happened". I was so embarrassed and felt like I could no longer fit in with anyone because I no longer had a mother.

Taking care of mom was a very traumatizing long journey that we never thought we would go through so soon. Each day we stayed busy doing something or had to go somewhere in preparation for the service. The next day, we met up with the funeral home directors to discuss arrangements, pick out a casket, and the way she would look. Dad, granny, Crystal, and I all knew momma was not a fan of make-up, so we asked if that could be limited. The mortician had made a disturbing comment and said mom's body was skin and bones, and that they would have to use special treatment to puff her body up. Dad told them to do what they had to but make her look good. That evening we picked her out a nice outfit, her favorite wig, some socks, and jewelry to help them get started. Later that week, dad received a phone call that mom was ready for viewing, so we all took a trip to see her. They did such an amazing job. She was beautiful and looked like herself! We were satisfied and ready for the hard moments to be over.

A few days before the wake, Crystal and I went shopping for outfits, got our hair done, something to eat, and back home. Dad then took us to Big T bazaar and had some t-shirts made with mom's picture. That night we got ready for the wake, and all I could think about was how I was going to hide my emotions the best I could. We arrived at the place and waited for everyone else to walk in and be seated. Watching people looking at my momma in a casket was another emotional trauma I wasn't sure how to deal with. We had so many people there that dad was afraid it wouldn't be enough space for as many folks mom knew, and he was right. A lot of people had to stand against the wall or wait until the viewing.

The next day at the funeral, there were so many people that you would have thought mom was a public figure or something, but she had a great heart and touched so many. Luckily we were memebrs to a two-story church, so it was more than enough space this time. Once everyone made it down the aisle to see mom for the last time, it was our turn. Dad, Crystal, and I walked up together and gave her one last kiss on the cheek. During the service, I slowly started to numb the feeling of pain because there was nothing more to say or that could be said to deal with the hurt we were in. I felt that since I still had dad, granny, and my sister that I could get through this, though no one thought I was hurting. I remember hearing someone say, "Brianna's not even crying" and "Brianna is holding it in," but I didn't understand why it even mattered to them. I guess if people didn't physically see the pain, that would make them think there weren't any, and if people did see the pain, they'd probably just think it was attention-seeking.

Halfway through the service, these dancing mimes came out and performed for my dad to a song called "After While" by Detrick Haddon. It was so soul touching that I burst out in tears after trying so hard to hold back. Once the funeral was over, most of the family and friends came back to our house for a repass. Everyone had smiles on their faces, talking, having a good time seeing one another, while I'm thinking about how life was going to be now that momma was gone. I felt so empty. Within the next few days, I had to encourage myself to go back to school. For my first day back, dad gave me a little pep talk to pray and ask God to give me the strength I needed, and I did. When I walked into my homeroom class, everyone stared at me from the door to my seat. My teacher kindly welcomed me back and presented me with some flowers and a bunch of sympathy cards from my teachers and all the 6th graders. It was really sweet of them because I know they didn't have to any of that.

About two hours into the day, I was sent to the counselor's office to what he was there for, but I quickly refused the help. I had silently developed the fear of what others would think of me. The following week, we received a financial gift from mom's job, and my demented self-snuck some of it to school the next day to buy my friends snacks out of the teacher's lounge. Towards the end of the day, I reached in my pocket and noticed my money roll was gone. I looked everywhere for it, and my friends helped me, but I had a feeling someone I knew stole it. I felt so bad and hoped dad didn't ask about it, because it was supposed to be in my piggy bank. Lesson learned.

CHAPTER FOUR

Waiting to Prevail

Mother's Day came on momma's birthday the following week, so granny, Crystal, and I went out to the gravesite to place flowers and balloons. What a way to spend the first Mother's Day without one right, but I'm so glad we had granny to lean on. Mom was the rock in our family, and the one who held everything together. When she died at the age of 34 it seemed like our whole world went into an abyss. We all knew we lost her in the years we needed her most, but we did well on doing what we needed to do to survive. Dad had seemed to be doing okay and taking things well, but he was also peacefully grieving. Crystal, however, put her emotional energy to use when she won a full scholarship after writing an essay on losing momma for a Susan G. Komen's Foundation contest.

On the other hand, I had to attend summer school since I couldn't pass any of my TASK tests. Upon my mother's request before she died, dad transferred me from Dallas to the Mesquite school district. At this point, I didn't see a reason to be excited about anything anymore, and the new school didn't even have a drill team.

One day, I was in my room getting things ready for the next day when I walked into the living room to get something. On the way back to my room, I glimpsed in the room momma died in, and scared the crap out of myself when I saw a figure that looked like her float across the room in a white dress. I quickly ran into my room praying out to God, to please tell my mom not to visit me that way anymore, and I never saw it again. The first day of 7th grade came. Crystal took me to school and walked me to class. Normally momma would walk me to class, but I was so glad my sister was there to comfort me.

That summer, Crystal had decided to go ahead and start her life by moving closer to her school, TWU, and her new job. In the meantime, dad had to find a new way to get me to school every day since his job required him to work early mornings. It was truly a struggle without mom, but one thing we never missed out on was a full cooked meal every night because dad was an excellent cook.

I began noticing that dad was giving a lot of his time to the computer, and I slowly figured out that he was online dating. Little did he know, I needed his attention more than anything. As time went on, I grew interested in things that would make me feel better or numb, like making dancing videos on YouTube, creating a My Space, and wanting a guy friend to love on. Right before my birthday, I created a sneaking habit, since Dad's favorite new word was "No." Of course, he wanted to protect me and make sure I didn't do anything I'd regret, but he didn't realize I was becoming anomalous. Later that year, he remarried an Asian woman who could not speak English and moved her into our house.

For my 13th birthday, I joined the step team at school, so I could deviate my mind from dad accidentally losing Fluffy when he went fishing one day. We looked everywhere for him, even posted flyers around our neighborhood, but no luck. I was forced to meet new people, and in the step team, I became close friends with a female I was finally able to relate to. We started riding to school together and going to each other's house.

I enjoyed the company so much because it took my mind off many things that she didn't know I was going through. The following school year, something came up, and her mom had to transfer her schools. I was lonely again until I met a new female friend who shared every single class with me during our 8th grade year. We started developing our likes for boys, and it was hard to get rid of. One day, I asked dad if I was allowed to have a boyfriend, and he quickly shot me down, saying I'd have to wait until I was 16.

That summer, I started going to Crystal's place to stay on weekends to get away and see how life was going to be out on her own. I was so proud of her because though I was the little sister, I still watched her grow up as well. I called her "the perfect sister," but she didn't understand what that meant. I always thought of her as perfect because she knew how to remain silent in certain situations. She always made smart choices and believed in herself to accomplish whatever her heart desired. A few weeks later she let the family know she was engaged. I was so happy that I shed tears because she deserved nothing but true happiness. Things were going pretty fast though because she found out they were pregnant with their first child a few months later.

My sister's passion was teaching, but it was also having her majorette drill team, which she started all on her own. I'd go support them during competitions when I could and would just be so proud of her for all her accomplishments. I knew I wanted to be around for my sister, and the new baby, so I started spending even more time with her. I'd even stay for weeks at a time with them. Some nights Crystal, and I'd be in the living room conversating about life, discussing wedding plans, or watch tv while I'd rub her belly because my niece would be kicking. Five months after my 14th birthday the baby was here! They named her Aliyah Precious after momma. We couldn't believe she wasn't here to share this wonderful moment with us. Then I started thinking about how she wouldn't be there for any future life events.

Back home things were crumbling, as I was finding myself in mild confrontations with Dad's new wife. To save money on the electric bill, she would cut the heat or air off during my crucial sleeping hours, which then produced a rageful spirit in me. As time went on, I slowly started to learn her ways and cultural differences from Americans.

She also wanted to become a nail technician, and I allowed her to practice with me. Her fried rice was also pretty good, and she was very smart about saving money. Dad ends up divorcing her a few years later. I guess he figured it just wasn't working out. Besides that, I was going through some serious emotional trauma. After explaining my frustration with dad, he began noticing the type of distress I was in and made me an appointment with a therapist.

A week later, after attending weekly sessions with my therapist, I realized that it wasn't helping me because I felt she couldn't relate to me being a young girl who lost her mom in the years I needed her the most. I explained to dad that I'd rather read the Bible and allow God to help me in my need for adversity. I had no idea why I said that and didn't know if I knew what I was talking about. When we returned home, I kept having the urge to pick up my Bible, so I went along with it. Unsure of where to start reading, I went to our desktop and google searched "why did my mom pass away bible scriptures." The first thing that stood out was "The Book of Job," so I grabbed my Bible and beginner reading Chapter 1.

For anyone that hasn't learned about Job, he was a wealthy man living with a large family and extensive flocks. God boasts to Satan about Job's goodness, but Satan believes that Job is only good because he was blessed abundantly. Satan challenges God that, if given PERMISSION to punish Job, he would turn his back on God." It was so interesting and detailed that I couldn't stop reading. After all the hurt, pain, and suffering he endured, he still trusted and followed God; he made Satan look like a complete fool. I realized that we can be honoring God, being a blessing to others, and it still rains on our life. What I took out of reading it was to always stay in faith, trust, and believe God no matter what storm may come. I felt like losing momma was a storm, but I knew now to continue to trust God and stay in faith.

The following month I was baptized at the Pathway of Life Church after accepting Christ as my Lord and Savior. I guess I thought I was supposed to walk away glowing or something, but I felt the same as I did before.

A month after my 16th birthday, dad, and I went to support Crystal as she graduated TWU with her teaching degree. We were so proud of her because though we went through a storm, God still gave her the strength to keep going. I remember as we grew up, we'd play "school" together, and she'd be a bossy teacher, even made me take naps! Teaching was something she desired doing, and she was able to accomplish her career goal by the grace of God.

CHAPTER FIVE

An Unconditional Healing

My basic sense of self hadn't sufficiently evolved into the years that were passing by, so I began seeing myself as having nothing to strive for in my future. I was two years away from graduating but had no clue what I would want to become in life. As the years went by I had a thought to become a social worker, until my history teacher commented that I wouldn't make enough money. I soon had a fanatical idea of becoming a mother, because I felt like the feeling would bring me such happiness. To get things off of my mind, I would go to my granny's house on the weekends, and also help babysit my niece. She was such a handful, that it curved my baby fever most of the time.

That summer, granny had been keeping a puppy that looked exactly like Fluffy, but he had a different color and mixture. She knew how much I missed Fluffy and let me take Charlie home to live with me. I was overjoyed and loved that I had something to love and take care of again. When I turned 17, dad broke the news to Crystal and me, that the house was being bought from the bank, and that we had a few months to move.

We were devastated, and in disbelief that we were losing the home we grew up in. Luckily, one of my brothers that were living with us at the time offered for us to live in a house he was getting built across town. It was bittersweet since I didn't want to move, but I also wanted to experience a newly built two-story home. There was one rule before moving across town, and that was to get rid of Charlie. Oh, my goodness! It felt like one punch in the face after another for me. Granny couldn't take him back due to living arrangements, so dad let my other brother adopt him.

In the summer of 2011, I received my driver's license after my dad placed me in a driving education course. That year I also had to replace my birth control. I had been longing for a baby again, so this time I invited God into the conversation. I asked God if he could allow me to become pregnant so that it be a boy to watch over his little sister if I was to ever have a girl. When it came time for the replacement, I had already planned things out with my then-boyfriend, who I gave no thought to think if he was ready or not. It wasn't long until I noticed weird symptoms and drove to the store to get a family dollar pregnancy test.

When I made it home, I quickly hid the test upstairs in my room and researched when it would be best to take it. The next morning, I took a deep breath, peed, and glanced down at the stick. Nothing had appeared so I waited, while in a panic state, and when I saw "positive" I was in disbelief, because I didn't think God thought it was time for me to have a child, but it was also what I prayed for. From many prayers I said in the past, this was his way of revealing to me that he does, and can bless us with whatever our hearts desire, but of course, that doesn't go for the doubters and unbelievers.

It was Sunday that day, so dad got my brother and me up for church, and I couldn't help but think through the whole service on how I was going to share this news with them, especially dad.   I texted both my sisters to tell them the news, and Crystal's first response was "Nooooo, make sure to see your ob-gyn to confirm". I did what she said. Our ride or die sister (Nicole) stepped in and took me to planned parenthood to confirm that I was indeed pregnant. The next day I went to granny's house to discuss how I should tell my dad, but I had to suck it up and just ask Crystal to be with me. He didn't take the news all that bad, but he was awfully upset at the choices I had made. He accused me of doing it on purpose, but I was too frightened, to tell the truth. The following week, my dad and I had to pull over into a 711 to call 911 after I developed severe abdominal pain from a cyst that was on my ovaries. It ended up being treatable, and we were sent home.

During my senior year, I had to be enrolled in a pregnancy care program that the school provided. My first three months were a struggle, but I was able to maintain myself, even at school. The baby's father and I were in separate districts, so we didn't see each other much. When I turned 18, I read in my bible Ephesians 6:1-3 "Children, obey your parents in the Lord, for this is right. "Honor your father and mother" (this is the first commandment with a promise), "that it may go well with you and that you may live long in the land." I realized being a disobedient kid would get years knocked off of my life. I came to my senses of how I misbehaved as a teenager, so I sat down with my dad one night to apologize for all my bad behavior over the years. He accepted and gave me an apology back.

A few weeks later I was given a large check amount from the SSI inheritance money momma left for me. It gave me a sense of security because I wasn't going to have to work right after the baby was born. Once we found out it was a boy, Crystal became so excited and started planning a baby shower. We had also been making plans for the baby and me to move in with her so that she could help in any way she could. I loved the idea, so I moved my furniture in while waiting for the baby.

On January 8th, 2012, Crystal and my niece were hit by a drunk driver that flipped and totaled her car. He ran and left them stranded at the scene. Thank God his hands were covering them because she was able to call for help. Two months later, we had a great "animals jungle" baby shower and received so much love from the family and friends that were able to make it. During the week of my due date, the obstetrician scheduled my day for induction, because my water had not broken on its own.

Crystal had hoped he didn't come on that Friday because she had parent-teacher conferences that night. I was in labor for 13 hours, and thirty minutes before he arrived, Crystal came through the door and was able to be by my side along with my baby's father.

April 13th, 2012 at 9:30 pm, Rafael Jr was born; with 3 strands of silver hair in his head, so I knew God made him special. While I was in the hospital with my baby, all of my friends were partying it up at the senior prom. At first, I hated that I missed it but didn't regret it one bit. I felt complete, and warm-hearted for the first time in years. Since there were only two months of school left, the program I was in, allowed me to complete all my classes through homeschooling. Graduation day came quickly it seemed, but I was ready to accomplish another great moment in life. I ended up not moving in with my sister due to a minor disagreement we had about the dad being able to stay some weekends to help care for the baby, but I still spent nights there.

I moved in with him, and his family, but still had to do my normal motherly routine. About ten months of an unsure relationship, I called my dad and let him know the baby, and I were moving back in. Without hesitation, he welcomed us back in, with open arms. I looked for a job, but I knew nothing about working. Yet, it was to the point that I ran through most of my funds because of my kind heart for helping others.

I found a small apartment not too far from my dad, and around the corner from granny, so I could help her whenever she needed it. I paid up my rent up in full and nailed my first job at Golden Corral as a host. It was a new, but fun experience for me, and I loved it. There was something about the feeling of making your own money, versus it being handed to you. Four months later I received an opportunity to work for the Post Office, but I was already satisfied where I was. I mentioned it to my dad, and he said "Girl, you better take that job, and make it a career."

I listened and went ahead to take the steps needed to be hired on with the post office. First I had to pay a $100 fee, then an 800-number called me for additional information. They let me know that after I passed a certain exam, I would be placed on the hiring list. I went to a private location to test, and I did great! I started my new position at the postal service after a three-month process. I then found out I was scammed into buying a position for the job, but I didn't even care, because I had gone from $7.25 to $13.75 within the first four months of 2013.

* * *

The night after my son's first birthday party, I had a dream that my momma came to visit and meet her grandbaby. She hugged us so tightly, and it felt so real that I was in tears when I woke up. I started spending the majority of my time at work, not realizing the actual time it was taking away from me being a mother. Since I was not permanent, we had to work serious overtime including weekends, and holidays.

I always stopped by granny's house the nights I'd leave work early. This specific night I received a message from Crystal that she was pregnant! I was so happy for them and prayed that this one was a boy for Jr to have a playmate. We started going to granny's every Sunday to spend time together and have a delicious dinner. Granny had magical hands when it came to soul food, and her amazing chocolate cake. Some nights I would sit and chat with her about life and she would say "Brianna, you think you're my age don't you?". I'd laugh and tell her, yes pretty much. I mean losing your mom at a young age will make you feel at least 45 by the time your teen years come.

CHAPTER SIX

A Beautiful Nightmare

During the first three months of Crystal's pregnancy, she had a very rough time dealing with morning sickness. She could be sick throughout a whole day. As the months passed by, she slowly started doing better, but would still feel a bit nauseated. I'd tell her "oh yes, this is your boy". When they went to find out the gender, she called me in excitement saying "It's a boy!" I knew it had to be, because of all the different changes she was experiencing this time around.

She ate healthy, took prenatal vitamins, and always listened to whatever her obstetrician suggested. She had been going to a church they joined in Desoto, Tx every Sunday and sometimes I'd join them. Our goal was to grow ourselves more spiritually in the word of God. A few months before her due date, our paternal grandmother who is also the family minister said the baby she was carrying was going to be an anointed child of God.

September that year, she hosted a beautiful "mustaches & bow tie" baby shower that I was happy to be a part of. I was glad because it was held before 5 pm, the time I always had to report to work. The following month her birthday came, but I was not able to make it to her "27th" gathering event and felt terrible about it since I had to work. By the time my 20th birthday came, Crystal would say she just couldn't believe that I was finally out of my teens. Three weeks later while taking her students on a field trip to the zoo, she went into active labor. By the time one of her friends got her to the hospital, she was already dilated to 6cm and had no time to get medications or an epidural. Three big natural pushes later, Christopher Jr. was born.

Two days later they were discharged and able to go home. As the weeks progressed, Crystal started feeling a bit weaker than usual and would have some minor trouble lying flat in bed to where she needed to prop up. Before her maternity leave ended, the principal asked if she didn't mind returning to work a little early. With my sister being the kind-hearted person she is, she said no, she didn't mind and made arrangements to return. During her sixth-week postpartum visit, she mentioned a few concerns to her OBGYN, who assured her that everything was normal. She continued to do her motherly/wifely duties and went through each day the best that she could.

Three months postpartum, and twenty-five days into 2014 while marching in the Martin Luther King Jr. parade, she suddenly felt completely out of breath and quickly followed her instincts to seek help. She drove to a local urgent care and could barely make it from the car to the office door without feeling so short of breath. When she finally made it in, the staff could see how in need of care she was and checked her vitals. She was told her oxygen levels were severely low, and she needed to be sent to the emergency room by ambulance immediately! She was beyond confused because she suspected it was only a cold but let them know she felt better driving herself. She called me saying she was on her way to the hospital for a suspected heart problem.

Once she arrived she was given immediate attention and underwent multiple testing. A few hours later a doctor looked over her reports and explained that her heart and lungs were completely covered in fluid. She was admitted overnight for additional testing, and they figured out that she was in full-blown heart failure. Yet they could not come up with a cause as to why.

When I made it to the hospital, I stormed in trying to figure out how professional physicians didn't understand what was happening to my sister. Crystal had to apologize on my behalf. I was in an emotional shock state, and in disbelief, with the information, we were receiving. They prescribed her medications, ordered a life vest (wearable defibrillator), and allowed her to go home after a week's stay. Getting used to her new food diet was a challenge, especially the days she longed for "Fried Chicken".

* * *

Now that I was living on my own, I had been praying for a guy to sweep me off my feet and love me for me. In my life, God never came in the times I wanted him to, but when he did, it was always worth the wait. A week later, my co-worker invited me to a BBQ, that I honestly didn't feel like going to. Then I thought instead of moping around, I might as well get my baby boy out of the house. Towards the end of that night, I was introduced to a handsome guy name Tech, who just so happened to be her older brother. We immediately fell for one another after a one-night phone conversation and moved in together two days later to begin our new relationship. The best part about him was having a job, being older, loving kids, and didn't have any himself yet which was the icing on the cake!

I had to have spoken too soon, because the following week he went to jail, lost his car, and his job that he'd been at for a while. I asked God if he was 'the one', but of course, I didn't receive an answer. But I did look at all the signs as a warning. He was gone for a week, and I fussed at him about warrants and anything else he had going on that needed to be straightened out. I was opening up to him quickly but kept my invisible wall of shield up too. As my sister continued to deal with complications in and out of the hospital, I told him I had a sister who I'd love for him to meet. We went to visit her, and I was so glad they met. My sister wanted to make sure he'd make me happy, so she questioned him on the spot.

Two weeks later, our granny, great aunt, and a few other family members put a delicious "bake sale" fundraiser together for her, and it was truly a blessing. We were raising funds to help increase her chances with being placed at the top of the heart transplant list. Each day that passed, she started having backaches caused by the life vest, but she continued to deal with it. Out of concerns for her keeping food down, and the cough that grew worse, she returned to the hospital. Later that evening they explained that her body was rejecting the medication. This meant that her heart was getting worse, and a heart transplant would be needed soon. It was suggested to her that a left ventricle assistance device (LVAD) would be able to give her heart a break, while she waited on a heart. She refused the option and stuck with the life vest that was still giving her back problems. One night I got off of work early and went to go keep her company. She was in pain, and her back was sore, so I told her to turn and let me massage where the pain was. She enjoyed that very much, and so did I.

Days would pass, and she would look at her phone wondering why no one was calling to check on her or come visit. I would uplift her the best I could and say "I don't want you to worry about anything we have no control over." In reality, I had no clue what she was feeling on the inside, but I always empathized with her when she would vent. I did let her know that whoever was meant to be around, that's who we'll go with. Even though deep down, it hurt me too.

We shared many memories, about momma too, and how she'd be causing hell trying to find out what's wrong with her child. It became silent for a moment, and she said softly, "This is not for me, this is for someone else". I didn't fully understand, but I told her that God had a reason for all he does, even if it's painful, which he's shown us before. At the end of that week, she was finally able to go home and be with her family.

She called and updated me one afternoon, saying "it's been two whole months, and there's still no match for a heart". I could hear in her voice the agony and concerning thoughts she must have been thinking. She said, "I just want to get better" and I said in a trembling voice "you will sis, I don't know what I'd do without you.". We both cried, dried our faces, and prayed. Some days later, Crystal had to go back to the hospital, and while there, the pastor of her church brought his family to all come to pray over her. They didn't keep her long this time, because we were told not much more could be done for her while waiting on a heart. She was discharged and sent home with an intravenous therapy (IV) bar. She had been continuing to read in her Bible as she was before the unexpected illness, but could not understand why her, and why now.

The month of April came, and though she was slowly losing energy by the day, she still made sure my niece enjoyed her 5th birthday. She also made it to her nephew's 2nd birthday. She was not allowed to drive, so she always had a driver if she went anywhere. One odd night, she dreamt her daughter said, "Mommy, Jesus is coming to get you". She took it as a sign or message, and began to prepare important paperwork, and even wrote sweet love notes to the kids, and her husband.

The following Sunday night, she texted me saying "Hey Bri, I may need you to take me to the hospital because I'm not feeling well again". I said, "ok sis, just let me know when to come". She replied, "well, I just called my nurse and she said it's best if I just stay home and come in the morning". I said, "ok, do I still need to come, I'll stay the night". She said, "no, my mom-in-law is here for now". I said "well, I'm going to check on you in the morning." We said love you and goodnight.

At 8 am, I got up and texted her because at this point she couldn't talk on the phone without constantly coughing. I said, "morning sis, you doing ok?". She replied and said, "yes, I'm feeling better". I said "good, just try to relax". I took a nap since I had to work that evening, but at 1 pm my granny called saying "BRIANNA, Crystal's heart stopped beating and she's being rushed to the hospital!" I immediately broke down, fell to my knees, and wanted to think the worst. Tech helped me get myself together and told me to get to the hospital. When I arrived, they had us all waiting outside the room she was in, while they got her placed on life support. I was curious to know what happened and asked her mother-in-law about it. She said, "everything happened so fast, we were sitting on the couch watching Judge Judy and then something quickly blocked my eyes, and when I looked up, Crystal was leaning over with her life vest going off". It took the paramedics a whole fifteen minutes to bring a pulse back, but I wasn't giving up hope for my sister.

She spent four days in ICU on the cardiac floor, and I went up there every day and sat next to her bed praying and singing many gospel songs in her ear. At one point, I thought she heard me, but she was no longer conscious. It was like I could feel God letting me know that I had to prepare for him to take her, but I just wasn't ready. Momma wasn't even here to help me through this double torture. I at least had daddy, both my granny's, and uncle's there for me. On the fourth day, all her organs started to shut down, and the doctor allowed us to see an X-ray of her oversized heart that was partially in her stomach. It was so devastating that the nurse shed tears, saying "27 was just too young to suffer from an unknown heart issue", and we agreed. On May 8th, her husband made the painful final decision. Everyone chose to stand outside to wait, but I told the nurses I wanted to stay by her side. The pastor's daughter who had been helping me coach my sister was very sweet to stand by my side. As soon as the nurse reached for the plug, I saw Crystal's hand move. I said, "wait! her hand is moving". The nurses both paused, looked at me, asked me to walk over and hold her hand to see that it was only the nerves. I went right back into my misery shell, while I rapidly watched her oxygen fall to 0.

The first thing I thought about after that dreadful moment was her and momma being together again because I know my sister missed her oh so much. All the family came in to say their goodbyes, and while I watched, it was like a momma situation all over again. I walked out of the room to find my grandma and ask her if it was ok to be mad at God. Because at that moment, I didn't know what to do, how to feel, or what was next. I heard my niece and nephew had arrived, and all I could do was hug them so tightly. Later that week we all met up at the funeral home to start arrangements, but I was not myself. I was there physically, but not at all mentally. I sent the funeral directors a picture of how I wanted her hair and was ready to bite anyone's head off whoever tried to get in my way on playing my little sister role. The next day her friends and one of our mom's friends had pissed me off after I walked into my sister's house with everyone trying to pick an obituary picture for her when I already had one in mind. I was ignored, wasn't listened to, and all the damn laughing nearly made me snap.

I got the hell up and stormed out to my car to call and cry to my granny. Leave it to her, she was able to get everything handled, and the obituary picture I selected was chosen. I understood that others didn't know what I was going through, but people needed to understand that someone grieving, no longer knows how it feels to not hurtinternally, impacting your sense of self, altering your priorities, causing emotional fluctuations like sadness, anger, and guilt. I pretty much stayed under dad, granny, and my baby boy, because I was now feeling the anxiety that grieving caused me. At the wake I just about tried to roll my eyes at everyone I thought didn't care, until granny saw me and tapped my leg saying "stop being like that Brianna." I don't even know how she was remaining so peaceful. After the funeral, I tried to hide my true emotions. It was devastating that I had to bury my sister on our mommas birthday. I was in a complete mental state. It's like after the burial, many people expect you to heal, and go back to life as normal. People say they'll pray for you, and meanwhile just thanking God it wasn't them. I developed a trauma loss syndrome after momma, and now I had to accept that God wanted my sister.

Over the next four months, I had been taking Jr (my son) to go visit granny on the weekends, along with my niece, and nephew who were there as well. In September I received a call from my uncle who was using granny's phone to call me, and he said, "Hey Bri, we up at the hospital with momma, she done had a stroke".

This was unbelievable, but I rushed to Parkland, where they were. It was a very long wait time, and before I had to go to work I walked with her to the restroom and chatted with her a bit to uplift her spirits. That night while I was working, my uncle called again and said granny just had a second stroke, and that it was worse than the first one. She now had some bleeding on the brain and could not move her whole left side. I remained in good spirits and told God to help my wounded heart because there was nothing good about this. When granny started rehab, I made sure I was able to come and attend a few sessions with her, since the hospital was close to my job.

I helped her eat, move, and even shower, but my goodness she was heavy! She was in the hospital for two months and was able to be placed in a retirement facility since no one could help her at home. I had never paid attention to the rumors about retirement homes, until I saw granny experience cold food, or waiting a long time for someone to take her to the restroom. Since I was there, I made a few complaints, but I was able to heat her food, and get her to the restroom on time.

On the weekend I started getting my niece and nephew more and would bring all three to see granny. It always brightened her day. A few weeks later, her health took a turn when the nurse staff noticed she was showing signs of heart complications. She was re-admitted into the hospital and remained there until she was stable again.

The doctor shared with us that her heart was not very strong, so in my head, I'm like how in the world is granny's heart weak. Granny then reminds us that after having my uncle (her 3rd child), she was told she had a weak heart, and not to have any more children. Well, it wasn't another child she had to worry about, but a stroke that resumed the state of damage. Before her stroke, we planned to go to one of her favorite casino spots when I turned 21, but now that was not possible, and I was sad about it.

Granny apologized for the state she was in and told me to go anyway and have a good time for her, so I did just that. I went to Winstar with only $60, lost it all, and went home broke. Sometime after New Year's I was going up the elevator to the floor granny was on and all of a sudden a faint feeling came over me. I quickly walked down the hall while my head was spinning, and as soon as I made it to granny's room, I laid next to her bed, held her hand, and the next thing I know, I woke up with her hand rubbing my head. I'm not sure what that was, but it wasn't the first time it has happened.

Later that week my uncle called our immediate family to come to get an update on her condition, and it was nothing I wanted to hear. The doctor said granny was not going to get any better at this point because her heart was too weak. That evening I went to chat with her about how she was feeling, and if she had any dreams of momma or Crystal yet. She softly said "Precious and Crystal came and asked me if I was ready, and I told them no, so they left". I knew once she said that it was very close to her time. I prayed to ask God to give me the strength to bear this type of pain again. I didn't know if the family was cursed or just had bad luck. I couldn't figure it out. The month of March came, and granny started to slip into a light coma, because she could still hear, but couldn't respond. I walked into her hospital room and talked to her like usual, but then I saw she was trying to snap out of her sleep. I said "granny you know God could heal you right now if he wanted to", and she scared the mess out of me because she fought through the coma and tried to sit up for 1 second but couldn't. I had never seen a reaction like that before. Before I left that day, I said "granny I love you, I know you hate this happened, but I want you to let go when you are ready, we will be ok, I will be okay, but I will miss you so much."

Two days later around 6 am, my uncle called and said "Bri, granny has gone." I pulled myself together, shed a few tears, and laid back down. I was confused, I felt alone, and I felt like I was next, even though I had developed my relationship with God. The next day I met up with my uncles at the funeral home, and of course, I picked the way granny hair would be, but they ended up having to cut it short, because of how matted it was from laying in the hospital bed. They still had her looking fabulous though.

I was sitting there on the front row seats again at a funeral, and I never felt so empty in my life. It was like that rage was starting to come over me again, especially after we buried granny next to mom, and Crystal. It was so nice of my dad to let granny have one of our family plots, so they could all be together. After that day, I didn't want to ever go to the cemetery again, because it was only one hole left next to them. From that day on, I felt like I was finally able to focus on building my relationship with Tech. Things even felt a little rocky with us due to how some of his family felt about me. I was going through such an emotional state, that if God wasn't walking with me, I probably would have gone seriously insane, or been in jail.

Months passed, and it was heavy on my mind to go dance at a club. See, I had gotten to the point where work was starting to feel like a place to go. Where I wasted 8hrs or more not being around my loved ones. I just wanted a way out, I felt so done with life and even told Tech that I was going to the club. It was kind of funny though, because back when Crystal was sick, I told her and granny I was going to go dance. After all, wasting time away from them was serious to me.

I ordered my pole, practiced with it, and even had one of my other sisters there to help me. We both sat down and plotted out business plans on creating a pole fitness studio and how we'll raise funds to get it. I knew I wasn't supposed to be there, but I was telling God how I just wanted to have fun in life. I made pretty decent cash but started seriously slacking at my original job. I spent two months there when a jealous dancer made up some nasty things about me, so I was terminated. I got in the car, cried from humiliation, and apologized to God because that was no one but him pulling my but out of there. I guess I wasn't realizing that the enemy was trying to tear me down little by little, especially after going through a back-to-back emotional trauma that I couldn't understand.

CHAPTER SEVEN

I'm Broken to Heal

Towards the end of the year, I had a feeling to give my baby boy a sibling, but deep down I knew I wanted to be married first and to make sure I did things right the second time. When the clock struck twelve on my 22nd birthday, Tech rushed out of the kitchen, got on one knee and proposed to me. He took the loaf of bread tie wrap, shaped it into a ring, and asked me to marry him. I immediately said yes, because why would I say no. What young girl that young didn't want to be married? Well, the one who didn't grow up with a mother, that's who. It didn't feel any different but calling him my fiancé instead of a boyfriend was the icing on my cake, aha! Our finances weren't so great, but I told him about my urge to want another baby. He mentioned that he always wanted a daughter but was never in a good position to have one.

Five months later on a Saturday, I woke up with a sore throat, sore breasts, and body chills. I woke my fiancé up and told him to take me to urgent care because I wasn't feeling too well. Once we got there it took at least an hour before I was called back, but after a urine sample, strep, and flu test, I was positive for strep, flu, and pregnancy! I was so excited and ready to share the news with my fiancé, who was waiting in the car. He was a bit nervous when I told him, but he was excited and hoping for a girl. When I got to week 9 I started feeling terrible and had a hard time keeping food down, on top of that I was already showing. Most days were a struggle at work with all the puking, and urinating, so sometimes I'd stay home or slack at work as much as I could.

I puked in the morning and I puked at night. I couldn't wait until the first trimester was over. A few weeks after entering second-trimester nausea did not subside, so I suffered daily. At the next prenatal visit, my obstetrician approved for me to take some over-the-counter medication to help with nausea. As the months passed, I started getting a little puffy in the legs, and feet, so my obstetrician said it would be best to stay off my feet as much as I could at home or work. The following month I enrolled my son into Pre-k and was blessed to have his grandma, and aunt help while I transitioned to a mother of two.

When I was 7 months pregnant, my amazing grandmother married Tech and me at the Fort Worth water gardens in front of our loved ones on September 24, 2016. We decided not to wait until we had the money to have a fancy wedding, and my father-in-law captured our entire day. Thanks to some family members who came up with a surprisingly beautiful, and unforgettable reception that evening. At the end of the night, we threw in a small gender reveal letting everyone know we were having a baby girl. Looking out at everyone without seeing momma, my sister, or granny had hurt me all over again when I was supposed to be enjoying my happiness.

A few weeks later, I slowed down going to work so much, because some days would be too exhausting, and I would have rather stayed home watching "love & basketball". The following month I had been feeling a flutter in my heart; something I never felt before. During the next prenatal visit, I asked my obstetrician to listen to it. She said I developed a small heart murmur that would go away after birth. After my 23rd birthday, I had dilated to 1cm, and it stayed that way until induction. Due to my water not breaking for the second time around, I was scheduled to be induced a day before my husband's birthday. The whole labor process was extremely stressful because the pain was horrible, I kept getting chills each time the anesthesiologist would insert the epidural, and then I was told I needed antibiotics due to being GBS positive.

After a rough thirteen hours, it was time to do practice pushes, but for some reason, my dilation didn't progress past 8cm. My ob-gyn explained that there was a lump in the way that was stopping the baby's head from passing through. I wasn't informed on what that was, so I didn't know what it meant. She did tell me that if I wasn't 10cm in 30 minutes, then she was going to prepare for a c-section. I prayed so hard to not have to be cut on, and when she came back she said let's try one more time.

All of a sudden my epidural numbness went away, and I was able to feel my babies head enough to push her out at just 8cm. It took up to thirty minutes for my placenta to be delivered, and I knew for sure this wasn't like the last time. I asked twice was everything alright, and she asked if I knew my blood type. Of course, I didn't, so she said not to worry about it. We welcomed our beautiful baby girl Talaycia La'Carroll, (named after Crystal) into the world on November 8, 2016, at 10:50 pm, on her daddy's birthday. My grandmother, cousin, and sister shared the moments in the room with us. My grandmother was a retired RN, and she noticed how much blood I lost, but she knew the ob-gyn would do her part, right.

Ten hours after labor I bled through five pads in 1 hour. I called in my nurse who said if I filled up another one to page her again. I got up to brush my teeth, then hopped in the shower where blood just kept falling down my legs. I stepped out of the shower, quickly grabbing some towels to wrap around my feet while I dried myself off and walked to the toilet. When I sat down to urinate I heard 3 big splashes fall in the toilet, so when I looked I there was baseball size clots in the toilet.

As I got ready to walk out of the bathroom I saw a black shadow pass the door. I immediately started praying to say God please, whatever that was I rebuke it right now! I kept telling myself that it was normal, due to this being the second time, so while my husband and daughter were sleeping, I was about to take a nap myself.

God put it on my heart to page the nurse before taking a nap, so I obeyed. Five seconds after she made it in to check my vaginal area, I began to faint. In the middle of me passing out, I kept hearing them talking and telling one another what step was next. The room filled up with a pool of nurses, but the main voice I heard was the anesthesiologist asking "who was her obstetrician", and "what's her blood type". He did his job so well; I was clapping in my head.

My blood pressure dropped to 60/40, and my blood count was at six. Moments later I was knocked out suddenly by the drug that killed Michael Jackson, called "the white". I was rushed into surgery where I needed four blood transfusions. It took almost five hours to stop the bleeding. During those five hours my dad was on his way to visit us. Tech called him and said I was bleeding too much, so they took me into surgery.

He got there as fast as he could, but it was only Tech and our baby girl in the room, without the mother. My dad assured Tech that things would be alright, but in reality, he didn't know what type of news they were about to get. My husband couldn't help but think, what if something happened to his wife, and how on earth would he raise this newborn child. After two hours, the nurses came to get the baby to help give him some time to himself. As soon as I woke up from surgery, the nurses came to explain what happened to me but didn't tell me why it happened. All I could think of was where was my family, and my baby girl. I wanted my baby girl so bad, that I was making the nurse sad to where she made them speed up the process for me to get a room. I felt like she was ripped away from me, she needed me every hour that I was away.

The next morning my blood pressure had a hard time going down. I also received news that my son was in a totaled car accident my blood pressure stayed up. I don't know what was going on in my life, I just wanted things to go how they did last time. We spent five more days in the hospital, and each day Tech would get off work at 3 am and come to take care of the baby. This gave me time to rest because I didn't want her in the nursery. All the nurses that came in loved her name, and one nurse loved it so much she wrote it on the board. I was enjoying being pampered, and having help with the baby, though she cried when others would touch her. Since I was there longer than normal, I asked the nurse if I could start pumping with their electric breast pumps for the preemie mothers. I was given one and made milk like crazy, nonstop. Even the nurses were amazed at how much I would make. They kept having to transfer my milk to the freezer section and would thaw it out before bringing it back for feeding.

The following day my ob-gyn came to visit me to make sure my uterus looked good, and before she left I asked her if she could check my heart, which was something she didn't normally do. An echocardiogram was sent up, and before I was discharged, I was told everything looked great. She set me up with a follow-up appointment with a cardiologist. When they called to make an appointment, I didn't see the reason to go since I was assured things were good.

For Christmas that year we went to my grandmother's, and my dad noticed that something didn't look right with me. At three weeks postpartum I had developed a horrible constant cough. I told him it was just sinus problems, so he gave me allergy medication. The pills never kicked in. When we arrived home, I could barely make it from the car to our front door; I had to pause halfway.

Once my husband helped me get in, I plopped down on the couch, because it felt like I just ran across a football field. I pumped milk later that night, and while doing so it felt like my heart was racing. I called for my husband to come to listen to my chest, and it sounded fast to him as well. We both connected it to just having a baby to keep from worrying. That night we tried to get intimate, but when I would lay flat it was a little difficult to breathe.

As soon as it was time for me to get in bed, I tried to lay down again, but this time it felt like I was underwater for several minutes, so I had to quickly sit up. The cough I had developed became very aggressive, so my husband slept in our son's room that night just to get enough rest for work. I was spitting up pink phlegm and gasping for air each time I tried to fall asleep. At four in the morning, I texted my dad and told him I couldn't breathe laying down and he immediately called saying that wasn't normal. He stated it sounded like pneumonia or bronchitis. He suggested

I go to the emergency room, but I told him I didn't feel that bad, and that I'll see my doctor later that week.

My dad wasn't hearing it, so he had me arrange proper care for the kids and came to take me to the hospital. I told my husband to go ahead and go to work, while the kids went to their grandparent's homes. When we arrived at the hospital, my oxygen level was at 82, and my blood pressure was 156/49. I immediately out crying because now I knew something was wrong. Unfortunately, due to a shortage of employees that day we were sent back to the waiting area until it was my turn to get an X-ray.

Two hours later, we were finally put in a room, but it took another two hours waiting for results. A doctor finally walked in saying my heart and lungs were covered with fluid causing me not to breathe. My heart was so enlarged that additional tests were ordered, especially after the doctor saw in my file that my sister died of a cardiac arrest with an unknown cause. I was asked to walk with a nurse to see how long it would take to run out of breath and it took only five minutes.

I was given this drug called Lasix that made me urinate all extra fluid from my body, causing me to lose forty pounds in one day. They then sent me for a CT scan and admitted me for overnight testing. That night I could not get any rest, because listening to my heartbeat while lying down caused some anxiety. I stayed up the whole time talking to God and praising him while playing my favorite gospel songs. The one on replay was by Yolanda Adams "This Battle Not Yours", then I instantly remembered Crystal saying "This isn't for me, it's for someone else". I wondered.

Overnight an echocardiogram was done, and throughout the night a nurse came in to weigh me. The following evening, a cardiologist named Michael Rothkoft walked into my room with his chart, already prepared to ask me every question he needed to make the proper diagnosis. He introduced himself and explained that my heart ejection fraction was functioning between 15%-20%. He said a normal heart function is between 55%-60%, and that mines were in the shape of an 80-year-old man.

He looked in my file and asked about my sister's situation, and after learning that she just had a baby as I did, he diagnosed us both with Postpartum Cardiomyopathy (PPCM). This is an often misdiagnosed, or unrecognized type of heart failure that occurs during pregnancy or later in the postpartum months. The condition weakens the heart muscle so that it becomes enlarged and can't pump blood properly to the rest of the body. He gave me a 50/50 chance to live. He ran my insurance to see all the available treatment options and ordered me a life vest – a wearable defibrillator. This was in case of a cardiac arrest, the vest would shock my heart back to life. It was only to be removed during a shower, and someone would have to be outside the door to hear if I collapsed.

The technician trained my son, husband, and me on what to do in case the vest ever went off. The vest was set to shock my chest if I ever went into cardiac arrest, but if anyone around me touched me while I was being resuscitated the vest would shock them as well. My son was only four at the time. He had to learn how to call 911 if I ever passed out at home, and to not touch me if it happened. My cardiologist set up cardiac rehab and told me to attend a heart failure clinic every week.

He also stopped me from breastfeeding, because my new medication would be harmful to my baby girl. So, the nurses and I spent all night squeezing milk out my breast due to them becoming painfully engorged from not pumping. I was given a hydrocodone pill to help with the pain, and they placed two wraps of towels around my boobs so the milk would dry. That night I tried to take a shower and ended up on the shower floor in severe weakness. I didn't have my vest on and knew it was very crucial to get back to it.

The bed seemed so far away from the shower floor, but by the grace of God, I was able to pull myself up using the metal rails. I finally made it to the bed, and my nurse who shared the same birthday as my son walked in saying "what are you doing Mrs. Harris?!". I told her I wanted to take a shower, but damn near fainted while doing so. I was completely naked, so she helped me get dressed, and explained that the side effects of the hydro pill made me react that way, and to not get in a warm shower after taking any in the future.

I was restricted from driving, working, and even eating certain foods with little to no salt. It was a struggle having a small support circle. So, getting back and forth to cardiac rehab was not easy. I thanked God for the loved ones he placed around us during an unexpected crisis. I was missing my babies so much, though they were in good hands. When my kids came to visit me in the hospital, I didn't know how life would go for them after this. I had to say goodbye each time I had a loved one in the hospital, but I prayed for a different outcome not knowing if it would be granted.

After a long week's stay, I got out of the hospital two days before New Year's. I was ready to start my new normal life, at least I thought. Between the medications, side effects, weakness, keeping track of my weight, eating the correct number of meals, and drinking a certain amount of liquid every day, it was all very overwhelming. Why did I think trying to survive would be easy, especially after being around it so many times before?

Two months later, due to me not being able to help my husband financially, we lost one of our cars and were forced to look for a new place to live after our landlord decided to no longer take our payment plans. I couldn't believe I was placed in the position to get a go fund me, but I had no other choice. We raised $1,300, and it was just enough to get us into our new place. Those people never knew how they saved us from living with other family members. Not many donated, but the ones that did, I sent a special prayer for them.

Living in today's world, income households are just very difficult, and this affected us emotionally, mentally, and physically as a couple, but God always made a way for us, no matter how sad things looked. One morning my husband received a job offer with great pay and benefits. This was a major blessing that came at the perfect time because he had just been let go from his previous job after being an hour late trying to take care of his family.

That same month, my nurses at rehab had learned that my sister died from the same illness and thought it would be a good idea to raise awareness for it throughout their hospital. They asked for my permission to contact their marketing team, and of course, I accepted but was in disbelief that anyone was interested in our story. I immediately felt like this was my moment. This was the moment I had been talking to God about those many years ago. I always knew I was unique, but never knowing my purpose of living through multiple tragedies. Through whatever, I knew to trust in him. I had faith even through everything always looked so upsetting in my personal life.

CHAPTER EIGHT

Every Reason to Praise God

In the midst of it all, God blessed me with a brave husband willing to walk by my side through sickness and in health, just like I saw my dad do for momma years ago. I was blessed with a handsome son and gorgeous daughter in the order I asked him for those few years back. This confirmed to me that he listened and was with me through every cloudy day. No matter who I thought I was, and what I thought I deserved, He was there.

The day we filmed the news segment, my cardiologist at Baylor Scott & White, told NBC 5 that they don't know what causes peripartum cardiomyopathy, but people who are African American may have a higher risk of developing the condition. Once our remarkable story aired, I was known as the patient celebrity in the doctor's office. Being through everything I had been through, it felt so good being welcomed that way. Many of my peers saw it as attention-seeking, but instead of looking at it that way I looked at it as a steppingstone; the same way I looked at my USPS career. A steppingstone to reach the main desires of your heart, becoming whatever it is that you feel you could be. Sometimes you get to a point in your life where you feel it's time to make a move, but not just any move because if not planned and done with God, it won't work out for very long. I learned that the hard way when he put me out of the club for trying to create the wrong business in my life. I remember the first day I met my cardiologist he stated that we were going to go off prayers and medication, so prayers and medications are what I went with, and it worked well for me.

The first three months after diagnosis, my heart function increased five percent higher than what it was. It was a miracle because I thought I was going to have to prepare to leave my babies and husband. My heart function was still at risk for cardiac arrest, so I had to continue wearing the life vest for another few months. It became so frustrating living with it.

Some of the worst moments with it would be getting intimate with my husband, hooked on doorknobs, and don't forget to set security alarms off when walking too close to one in the grocery stores. Sometimes I would think about what if my heart stopped while in public, or even while holding my baby girl in my arms. I talked to God so much, that if he were still human he probably would have sealed my lips.

Honestly after so many heartbreaks, and having a broken heart, all I saw was him. I bonded with my little family as much as I could, and we were able to make it to church most Sundays with my parents-in-law. Between them and my dad, Tech and I were able to stay afloat and continue to rebuild ourselves up. Although I liked getting out of the house, I would be embarrassed walking around with the vest, because wondering minds always had questions.

Three more months had passed, and my heart function was still at risk for a cardiac arrest, and due to my sister dying from one, my cardiologist let me know that it would be best to get an implantable defibrillator. He explained that my second cardiologist would go in to make a pocket above my heart to place the device. There were pros and cons to it, but I had no choice but to accept whatever I had to do. I asked him if I was able to return to work part-time, even though I still had my life vest on. He approved it, and when I returned to work everyone welcomed me back with opening smiles, hugs, and a card filled with donations.

Two weeks later I received my implantable defibrillator and had to take some time off again. It was a lot better than carrying around my life vest, which I had to mail back since I didn't need it anymore. One night Tech and I were sitting on the balcony talking about our past. As soon as I brought up Crystal's name my eyes went blue, and I immediately couldn't breathe. My husband carried me to the couch, and I told him to call 911 because my heart would not slow down. When they arrived, my body calmed down, and they let me know that talking about my sister triggered a severe anxiety attack. My heart rate was rapidly increasing which wasn't good in my case because the defibrillator will shock me if it reaches a certain level. I never knew anxiety was real until that frightening moment.

Upon my return to work for the second time, I started getting treated certain ways by co-workers who had been there for years, because they didn't like that I was placed on light duty being so young. A lot of people still didn't know my situation, and that was fine with me until I started being asked to do things against my restrictions. I showed my scar and lump every chance I had to show them I was not to be played with. I was now covered medically and given time off when needed. I used this time to brainstorm about if I continued to get better, what would be the reason I went through all of this. I knew it couldn't be just returning to work, acting as if my life wasn't at risk months ago. The following year, I randomly looked up my condition on Facebook, and all of a sudden these support groups popped up, leaving me in total shock! I couldn't believe there were others like my sister, and me. I joined the most followed groups and began sharing my story.

In the group we were called "heart sisters", so I thought of creating a short film for all the local ones to publicly raise awareness. Only three were able to be a part, but it still went amazing. On top of that, I had some family and friends join in on my special project which led to success. So, I quickly started thinking of more things that I could be doing to raise awareness. On September 30, 2018, I was at work when I all of a sudden heard God ask me what I was waiting for, so I responded in my head saying "God I have no funds or time management for it." Then he said it again, "What are you waiting for." I literally stopped what I was doing, grabbed a pen, some paper, and started writing nonstop, daily.

I thought of "LetsTalkPPCM", because if only someone would have talked about it, maybe my sister would be alive today. I started reaching out to many women who battled with Peripartum Cardiomyopathy (PPCM), is an often unrecognized form of heart failure that occurs during pregnancy or up to 12 months postpartum. The condition weakens the heart muscle and causes the heart to become enlarged. As a result, the heart can't pump blood properly to the rest of the body. A pregnancy induced heart condition that and asked if they'd like to be added to my blog page. I would be ignored, get some no's, but the ones who were willing to help were a blessing. It's hard trying to remember certain traumas that happened in our life, but the worst part is acting as if we've never experienced it.

That year for Thanksgiving, we were able to plan a relaxing getaway cruise vacation to the Bahamas alongside my husband's parents. The kids had such an amazing time, and my husband enjoyed it more than them. Creating beautiful memories with my kids has always been my number one priority, and I was glad it was finally starting. A month after our trip, we received a devastating phone call that my father-in-law suffered a massive stroke and did not survive. It was very difficult watching my husband go through an emotional trauma I knew about all too well. I then realized that I was not able to help him grieve since I never fully healed from the deaths of my loved ones. Two years after diagnosis I was considered fully recovered, and my cardiologist called it a spontaneous recovery.

* * *

I had a co-worker who approached me at work one day, telling me that her daughter needed patient advocates to speak at a "Delta Tea Meeting" that they host every year. I felt honored and immediately accepted to be a part of it. I knew then, this was God confirming to me that I was going in the right direction. Her daughter and camera person had to come to interview my husband and I, but when it came time to present my story, our video had some difficulties, so we never saw it. I was saddened by it, but grateful that I was able to share my story with over one hundred people that I didn't know. Out of nowhere, I was approached by a lady who said she used to work with my sister, but never knew what happened to her. She gave her condolences and took a copy of the obituary I had with me.

A few months later, God placed on my heart to go begin to form a nonprofit organization, and not to worry about the money I would need to spend on it. I did exactly that. By the end of the year, I received an email from a reporter at "Pro Publica" who was interested in learning about my story. A month later, the founder of a Texas organization called "MoMMAs Voices" emailed me to come to share my postpartum hemorrhaged story that led up to my heart condition. Two months into the year 2020, I was asked to become partners with that same organization to be soon placed in rooms with actual healthcare providers.

It was funny, because I had been reaching out to others who were ahead of me in the business process, but it was impossible get help from people who only saw me as competition. I was so happy God sent someone willing to give me a chance to help touch and save many lives like I knew I could.

During February's heart month, I put together my first awareness music video that would bring in a unique way to spread the word. That same month I was invited to the "40th Annual Meeting of Advancing Pregnancy Research" event, and it was beautiful! I met more of my colleagues that were connected under MoMMAs Voices, and one of the ladies there fell in love with an awareness music video. She recommended my name to an organization in California that she was telling me about, and the lady responded saying she would be in touch with me. That summer I partnered with the California team. Two months later some representatives from the American College of Obstetrician & Gynecologist

(ACOG) emailed me after being given my name from a doctor in my California team.

At this point, I was overwhelmed but had to remain focus on the bigger picture. Which was everyone was interested in my story, and that God was making it all come together. I even had an interview with The Press Association in London, UK who published my story in their news article.

We were all in the middle of a pandemic dealing with Covid-19, but that didn't stop God from walking with us. When I heard about the stimulus checks I automatically knew God was up to something. A drastic change was coming that was going to be good for some, and bad for others. I suddenly started experiencing body pains and begin to complain to my doctors about it. The good news was that it wasn't heart-related, so my primary care physician suggested it was job-related.

The pain would start at my toes and work its way up to my shoulders on both sides of my body. Each day became more of a struggle to get up for work. The days I did go, it would be difficult for me to stay awake around 1 P.M. every single day. Thanks to covid, I was able to take some time off work to care for myself, and the kids as they learned to live a temporary new life. The worst part about it was wearing masks everywhere and working for 8 hours with one while already dealing with bad anxiety.

I went through months of testing, but nothing could ever be found on the cause of the pain. After multiple doctors' appointments, I was finally given the diagnosis of Fibromyalgia. Fibromyalgia is a disorder characterized by widespread musculoskeletal pain accompanied by fatigue, sleep, memory, and mood issues. Researchers believe that fibromyalgia amplifies painful sensations by affecting the way your brain and spinal cord process painful and nonpainful signals. I know right? What a horrible condition to develop after heart troubles. I could've let it keep me in distress, but 1 Corinthians 10:12-14 says "No temptation has overtaken you except what is common to mankind. And God is faithful; he will not let you be tempted beyond what you can bear." I

The holidays were extremely different since no large family gatherings were happening, but my little family, and I enjoyed it. The kids even had the best Christmas ever that year (in their words). In my mind, I knew it was all a part of Gods plan. There have been many times where people would ask how I knew it was God talking to me, providing for me or how I was able to hear him though he had no voice. I tell them that somewhere between God showing me that dream at seven, taking my mom at twelve, and going through a severe state of grief, it all led me to pick up the Bible three years later. I used to think that you had to be an old person just to experience God, but he showed me otherwise. When my sister became sick, she felt that it was not for her, but someone else. She was right, and I wanted her to know that so badly.

Three months later while taking a power nap, God sent Crystal's voice in a dream, basically a phone conversation with one another, but it felt so real! Before I woke up, I said "Crystal you'll never believe what they said I have", she said, "Yes Bri, I know. You have what I had." That was the strangest dream ever because she never found out why her heart failed. It was like God was letting me know that she was happy, healed, and well. God always had a certain way he would send me answers, confirmations, or reminders like that for me. I learned how to catch on by reading certain scriptures in the Bible that would apply to my life.

When I found out about granny's stroke I was so confused as to what my family had done to deserve back-to-back illnesses. Once she passed away, my uncles, cousins, and I had to remove all the items from her home. We were all taking things we wanted to keep in her memory when my uncle picked up the VCR and hit the eject button. An old video of Crystal's seventh birthday had been playing recently. I knew then that granny passed away from pure heartbreak. She had to bury her mother, daughter, and now the first grandchild so I could only imagine how life was feeling for her. The sad thing about grief is that no one else will care about it, as much as you do. Especially if they have never experienced the heartbreak of back-to-back trauma. My happy place was dancing in my head and seeing mini visions of myself doing things I always dreamed of.

* * *

I never knew about generational curses until I came across them in the Bible one day, not because of what someone told me. Some non-believers think the Bible was edited, and yes it probably was, but the way of living can still be found in it. There are a lot of uneducated young people out there who are only being placed in front of sinful situations. Not many people are thinking about how their kids are having to survive right along with them if poverty is involved. I always told myself that there has to be away out of certain situations that make us unhappy, depressed, angry, envious, confused, or even exhausted. I think somewhere on this journey, God is going to have me speaking for him, and one of my first cousins on my dad's side proved it. At our family function in 2019, she said "Bri, granny told me to tell you this. I had a dream that you were standing in front of thousands of people speaking about God". I couldn't believe what she had just told me, but I took that word and received it down in my spirit!

January 1, 2021, God revealed to me that I was finally prepared to write my first book, not just any book, but my actual story. He wanted me to share this heartbroken story with others who may need the knowledge on how to surrender and receive God at a young age. I found some healing in my storytelling when I realized it was interesting to others who never met me a day in their life. Sharing my story without a book alone, proved to me that this was indeed a gift I should jump on. I prayed on it and set a goal to write my book in three months. The first week of writing, I started with three pages a day, but then I started slipping away from myself. I started slacking at work, and my body would ache more, causing my hands to flare up in pain. I should have seen a distraction coming because as soon as humans try to make a change in life or make a good decision that can bring about change to their life, the enemy goes and get permission from God to tamper with you. We are often not taught as children the importance of learning about Jesus and how he died to save the entire world. It sounds unbelievable sometimes, or too good to be true, but once you give your heart to God, and admit your wrongs then he will open your eyes to so much more than what you thought you could see.

I often wondered, why is it that when we're young we're exposed to so many different chapters in life like abuse, drugs, addiction, loss, traumas, etc.,. Yet as soon as we're older whichever chapter we went with will determine the way we stumble in our purpose. Most adults forget to teach their children that they can become whatever they want to be if their heart desires it. Never ruin a child's dream or ignore their true feelings in any situation unless they are completely in the wrong. Whooping's help sometimes at a certain age, but once they're older, what are you going to do then? become rebellious to the child, or try to numb your love for the child, all in the acts of what the enemy wants to make happen. He wants more kids lost in the world so that they would never find the purpose God has for them.

People will tell you that only money can make their situation better, but is that true? I answered my question when I ran across Luke 16:13 "No one can serve two masters. Either you will hate the one and love the other, or you will be devoted to the one and despise the other. You cannot serve both God and money." As it came closer to finishing my book, I finally understood what was taking me so long to start it in the first place. It was the pain that brought back so many memories I once put in numbing boxing.

The numbing box is when humans go through a difficult trauma and try to remove the true emotions of self and place them in a numbing box. As life continues to happen God is constantly molding you, and the emotions that are in that box will be tested. In my life, he knew what could ruffle my feathers, and also what could bring out the best in me. Strengthening me, guiding me, and molding me into who he already knew I would be one day.

My husband and I were fortunate to still have our jobs after 2020, so we chose to invest the spare funds into educating ourselves. In between times, my son became a virtual learner, and my daughter adjusted to having to wear a mask over her face in public. Life was beyond different than what we were used to, but that's how God gets our attention best. I started small therapy sessions at home with the kids, and my husband to make sure we were all remaining sane.

This opened up certain topics that a home would benefit from in times like today. I sat the kids down one day and told them I want them to write about whatever they want. Talaycia made a book on how she stole momma gummy bears, and Rafael wrote on his transition from public school to virtual. During this moment, God revealed to me that I had little entrepreneurs on my hands and that they too can become whatever they wanted to be in life, as long as He was in the middle.

* * *

Since I was a child, I was disliked by my dad's other children for a while. I never understood why until I was older to notice that their feelings were shattered as kids. I would lose friends at school over liking certain boys, or if I didn't fit in the way they wanted me to. I had many family members who looked at me funny because my dad always had my back no matter what anyone else thought. A lot of people grew to dislike me before I was able to reach my purpose, and now I finally see why. Once God starts to elevate you, He will open your eyes to things you may have not paid attention to before.

He opens your heart and mind to discerning others around you and may even give you a warning. If someone has ever been envious of you, unhappy with you, unforgiving to you, unfaithful towards you, or anything in the negative we still have to love them and forgive them, but never force ourselves to keep them hanging around to do it again. Luke 6:27-28 Jesus said, "But I tell you who hear me: Love your enemies, do good to those who hate you, bless those who curse you, pray for those who mistreat you".

One of the main things I've always struggled with was forgiving people who wronged or caused pain in any way towards me. I was the hurt person who enjoyed hurting others because it felt better. No one understands what a person that's living that way is going through each day. People snap and end up going insane over some of the things I already experienced in life. It's amazing how God works because though He knew I was this sad, angry, and hurt young lady, He still decided to place a drive down on the inside of me.

Everyone has that moment in their life when it's time to take that step, and this was my time. I decided to be that young, African American lady to allow God to use me in every way I could be used. I owed him that, and so much more for sparing my life to be here today. I pray that everything my heart desires will be accomplished before the day I leave this world to join my loved ones.

CHAPTER NINE

Life on Pause

The purpose of my life was already set in place the day I was born. I always thought being my dad's very last child was weird, but I never thought my story would be remarkable enough for others to enjoy and heal from. I tell others all the time now, that if someone would have just shared their heart failure story with Peripartum Cardiomyopathy then maybe my sister would've had the chance to live, be here for her babies who miss her dearly.

I never had a doula, but in 2021 I wanted to become one to further my education on how I Observed at childbirth. I didn't have the funds at the time, so I was going to hold off on it like I always do. Out of nowhere, one of my amazing heart sisters reached out to ask me if I still wanted to doula, I told her yes! She gifted me with a training class that was approved by a popular doula organization. If only I had become one before my sister's heart failed, I could've known the warning signs that would have saved her life. I held on to the pain of both her and momma so strongly because no one understands that they were all I had growing up and being around them at any gatherings. I no longer enjoy gatherings as much or getting to know other family members who weren't around, to begin with, and if they were, I wouldn't remember them.

When I was twelve, it felt like life had stopped for me, losing my momma trapped me in a world of grief-trauma that I was unaware of for many years. I secretly believed that I'd never be anything in life since she was gone. I had to be raised by my dad which had some very difficult moments. Like when it came time to buy sanitary napkins or explaining my true feelings and emotions for guys. I didn't know how to become a young lady after my sister moved out, so I brought attention to myself the best I could. My dad did everything right in the way he knew how to, but he didn't know how badly affected I became after momma passed away. It wasn't until after learning to grieve the loss of my sister and granny that made me realize what I'd been dealing with all those years.

Paused in a moment that I could not re-do or take back was heartbreak on top of more heartbreak. Everyone's relationship with loss is different, and therefore everyone's grief experience won't be the same. Someone may be struck with heavy grief at the loss of a pet that played a very significant part in their life. Whereas others may not mourn the loss of an estranged parent. We had a family dog I grew up with name Rocky, and when he became old and developed cataracts I went insane, especially after my dad decided to put him down. In my young mind, I felt so extremely hurt, because I had an attachment with him. There is no right or wrong way to grieve. Some may become violent, sad, mentally ill, or in rare cases may be satisfied the person is gone.

Over time I've learned that grief may be accompanied by a range of emotional changes including sadness, guilt, anger, relief, joy, isolation, or even numbness, particularly if you had an ambivalent relationship with what was lost. It is also common to cycle through these different emotions at different times. You may develop insomnia where you find it hard to fall asleep, or stay asleep, which is common in those going through a grief experience. Lying in bed feeling overwhelmed by emotion and memories can have a real impact on your sleep, let alone your social life. While I was going through my grieving process to prepare for my sister, and granny to transition I hated the fact that I still had to report to work. I hated that to make money mean I had to spend daily hours away from my loved ones. I hated that I had blown through all the money my momma left, and I hated that I didn't feel smart enough to accomplish certain goals. I was lost in the world of grief, and it's sad to say that some people rather see you that way.

Some grievers develop hallucinations and may hear the voice of a deceased loved one or seeing their image can be very common in the grieving process. For many, the intensity of grief will fluctuate over time, increasing around significant moments such as birthdays and anniversaries, life events, because these types of moments in life hurt all over again. My mom missed my high school graduation, her daughters becoming wives, and mothers, being a wonderful grandmother, and just being there to hold on to. Looking for a mother in other women became impossible, so I knew not to become too attached to certain women. God would place many experienced individuals around me to teach me in my observing season. My sister isn't here to enjoy her babies and be able to enjoy her career she worked so hard for. My granny didn't get the chance to take me to the casino we always talked about doing, and the fact I could no longer go visit with her every Sunday to eat or try on all her perfumes was truly depressing.

Receiving a significant health diagnosis for some can mean making positive lifestyle changes, but for others, it can be a loss of quality of life and may also result in a loss of social connections. As you can see, losing someone or something can mean different things to different people, loss of routine, loss of identity, loss of hopes and dreams, loss of quality of life and social connections.

Family members are trying to figure out why I'd rather not be around them or attached to them, and that is because my family is never talked about, almost like they never even existed. I still deal with my difficult past moments, but I continue to go to God for all my healing, and peace that I need. Every time I pray for peace, it's like a warm coat God places over me to calm down.

Grief for the death of a mother is one of the hardest things we face in life, but nearly all of us have to face it at some time. Everyone's grief is different, and we all have our ways of coping. We may feel some or all of the emotions of grief at times, or we might just feel numb and blank. I was numbed for so long after my mom's death that when I finally realized it, I was a total pain in the ass for others. Some people, for various reasons, may need some more professional guidance if they get paused in their grief or don't have any close support that can relate. It was extremely hard for me to continue to push through life as if I wasn't hurting. Being in your teens you just want to keep up with the rest of the group, not spend it crying and being sad all the time. I didn't understand that not having friends that related to my trauma affected me.

I thank God so much for where I am today. Though He might not have blessed us with a pocketful of cash, He's blessed my little family with love, and more time to spend together. I became big on teaching them about Jesus, prayers, and dealing with their emotions the proper way. I grew to learn the hard way that family doesn't always mean "love" or "will always be there". This was something I knew for sure to teach my children, niece, and nephew. You'd be surprised at how people feel about you while watching you go through a traumatic experience. I once read that "There are some people that will know your struggles, your pain, have seen you cry, have evidence of your past, or even know your secrets. They don't like the fact that other people see you victorious! When others see a smile on your face and compliment you on being strong, it probably makes their ears bleed. These people hate it so much, that they talk about you every chance they get. They can't be happy for you, and definitely can't celebrate with you. They may have more than you, but envy everything about your spirit. They're envious of your win with God because that wins money can't buy! I hope you continue to let your light shine, know that you are here for a purpose in your life."

I'm praying that God blesses whoever may read this book and that you're blessed with all your heart's desires, and that's for your children, your children's children and for many generations to come. The world is full of strangers, waiting to root for you, and all your amazing accomplishments! Write the book, tell the story, help heal a child or even an adult. We are all brought to earth to be broken and healed for others once finding our purpose.

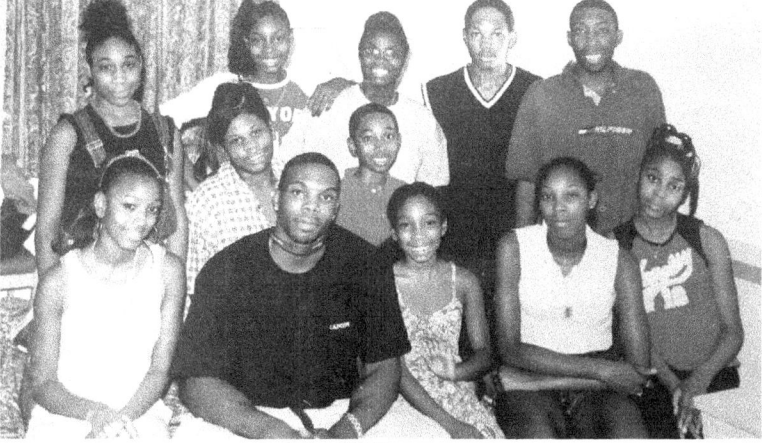

My Siblings

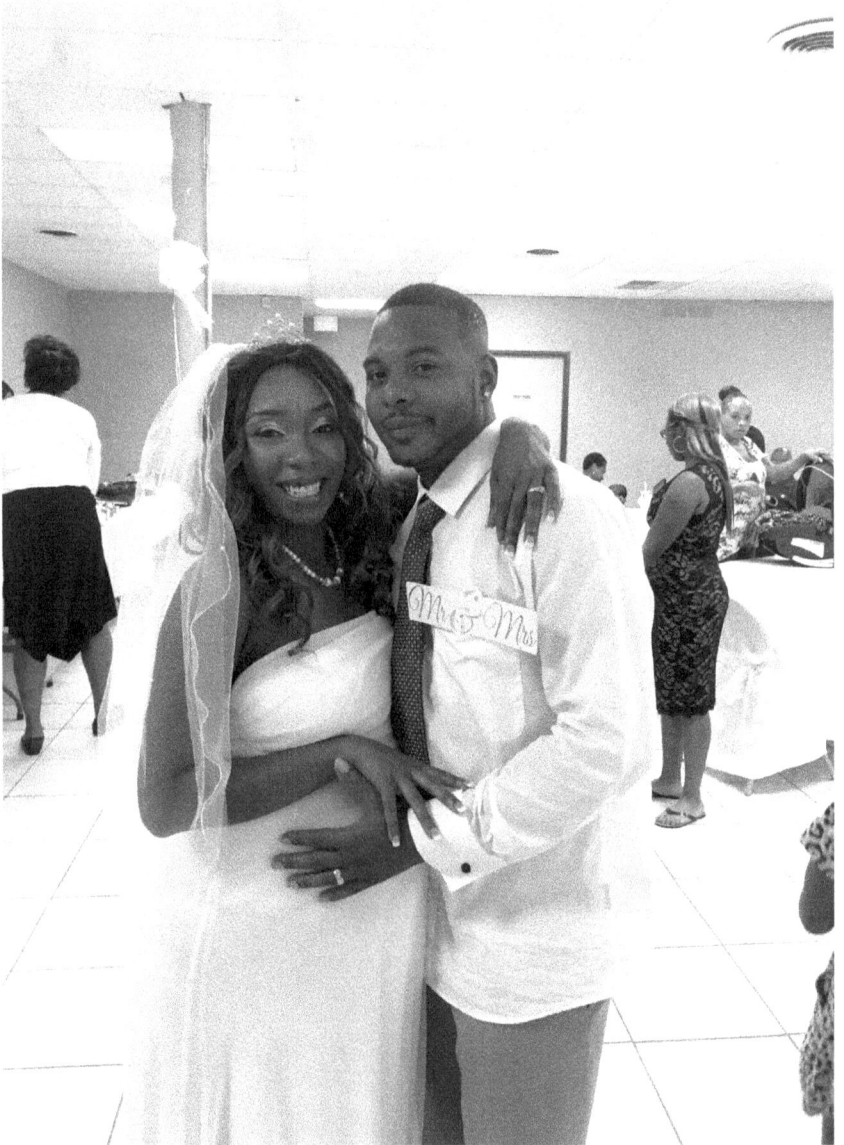

My husband and I at our wedding.

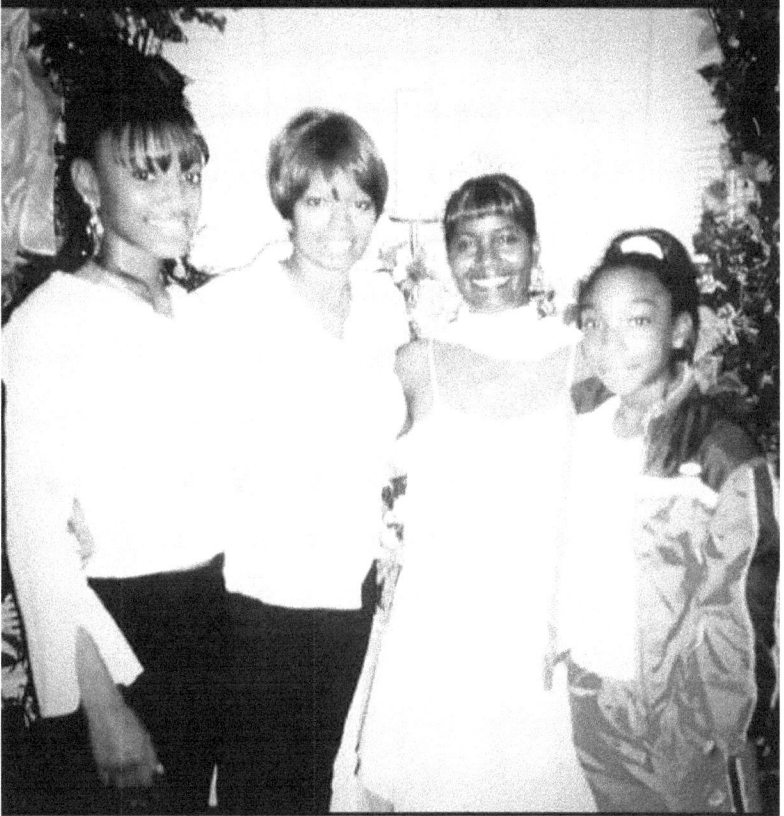

A Family photo with Crystal(sister) on far left, Precious(my mom), Carol(My Grandmother) and me on the far right.

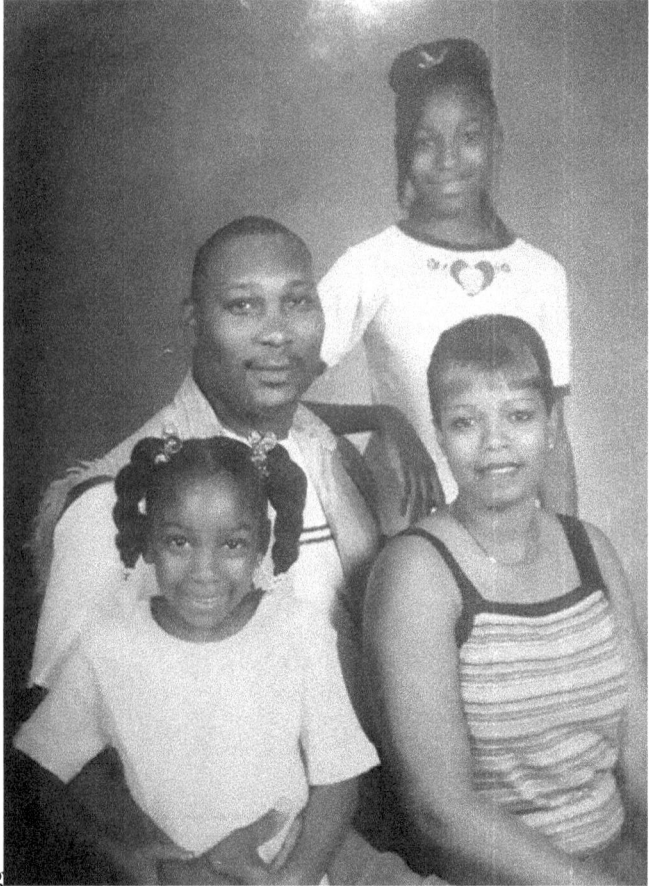

My Mom, Dad, Sister and I.

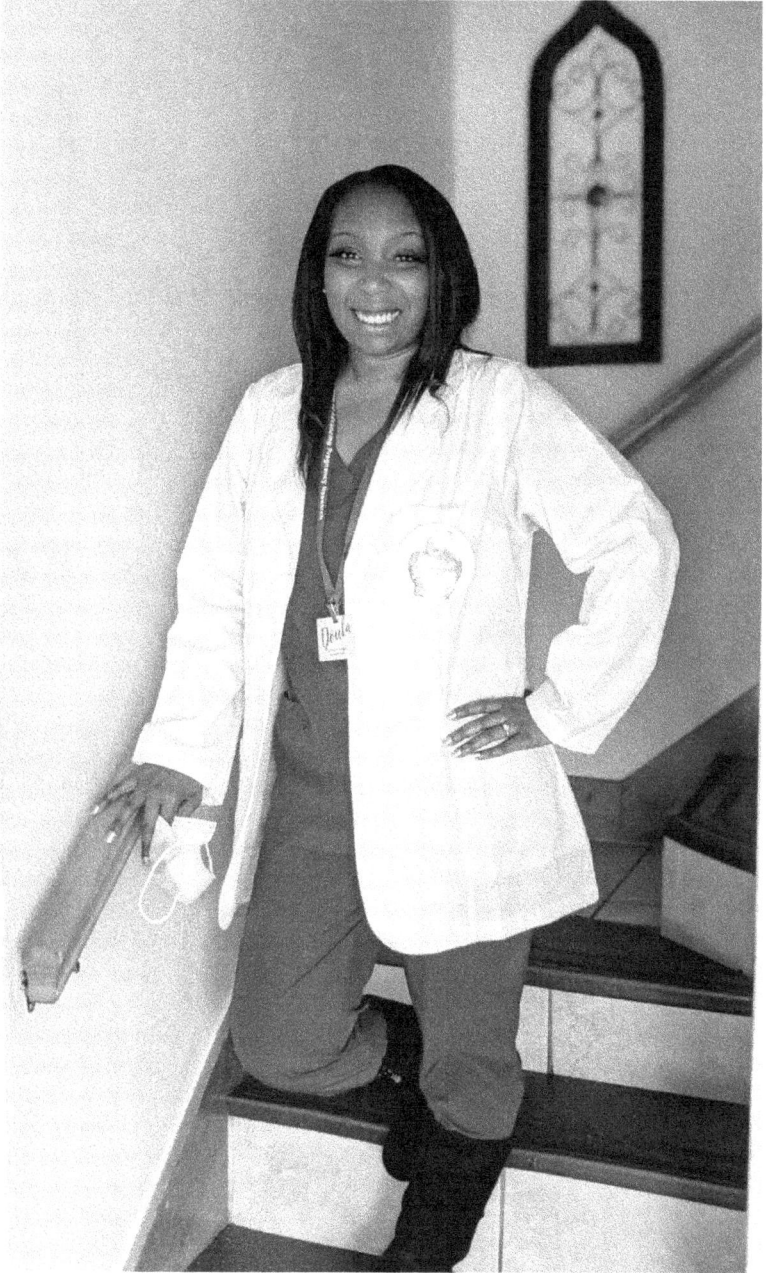

I am now a doula.

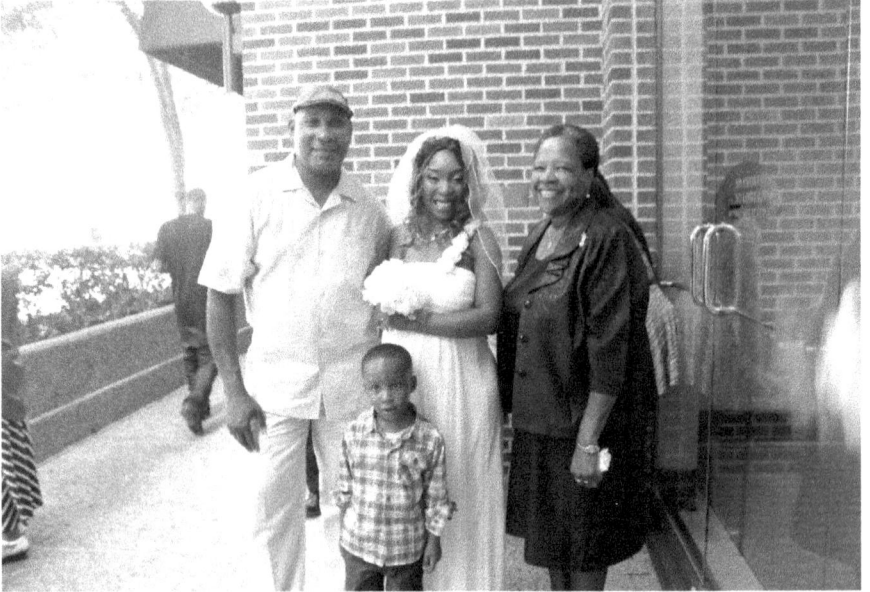

Paternal grandmother (Peggy), my dad (Ricci), and Son.

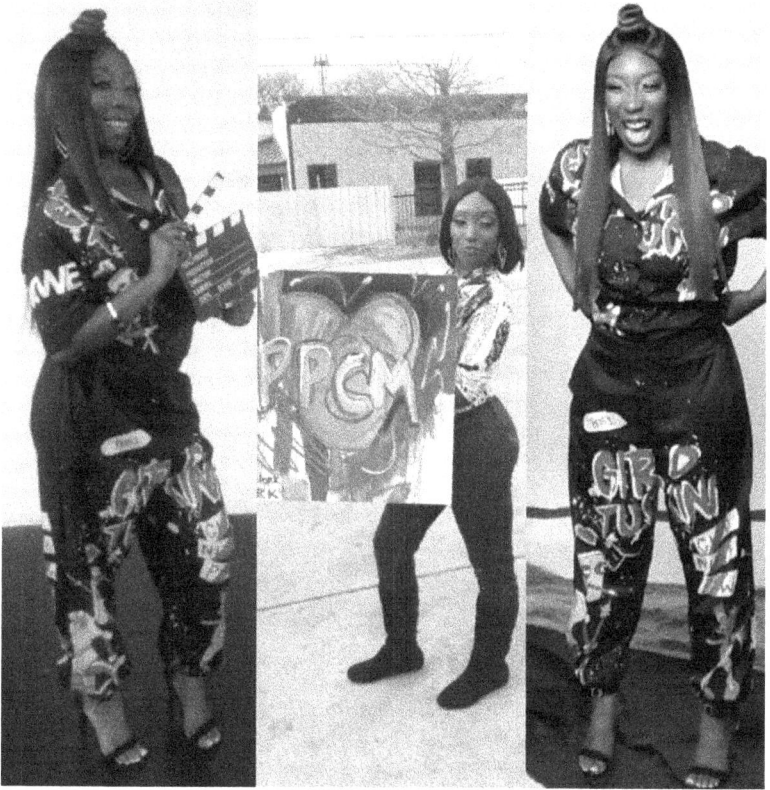

Increasing awareness with music and films.

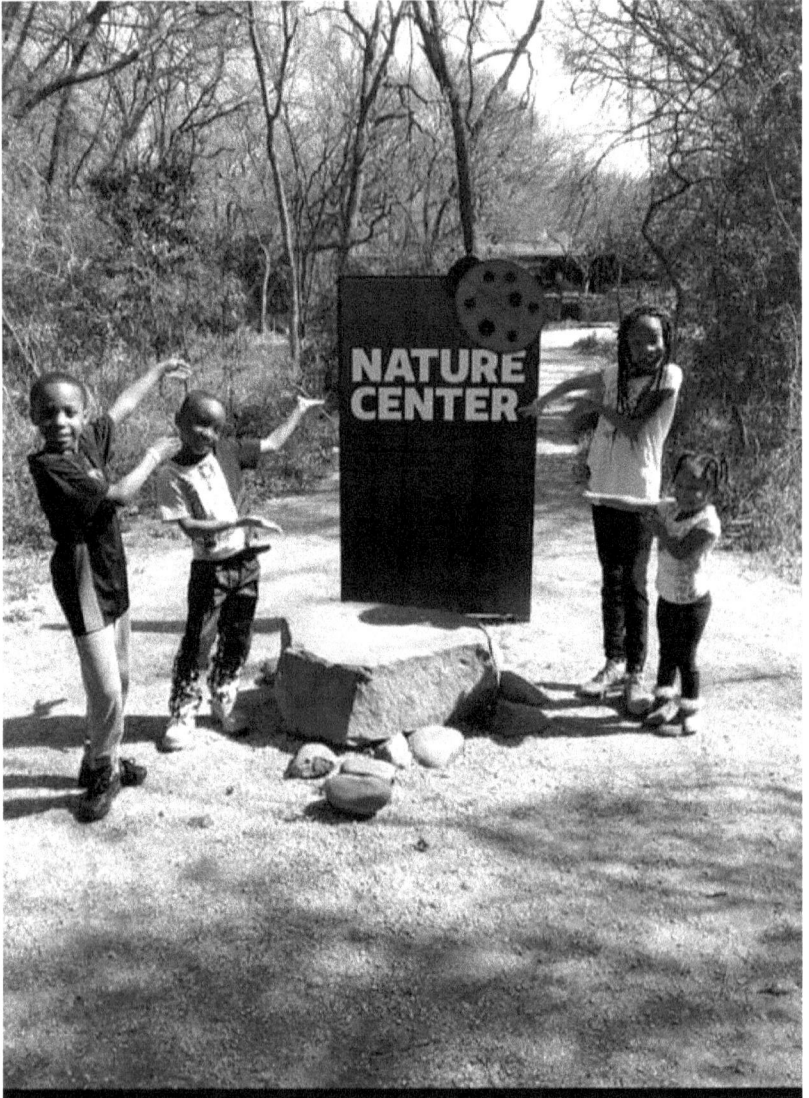

A photo of my niece and nephew with my kids at Nature center.

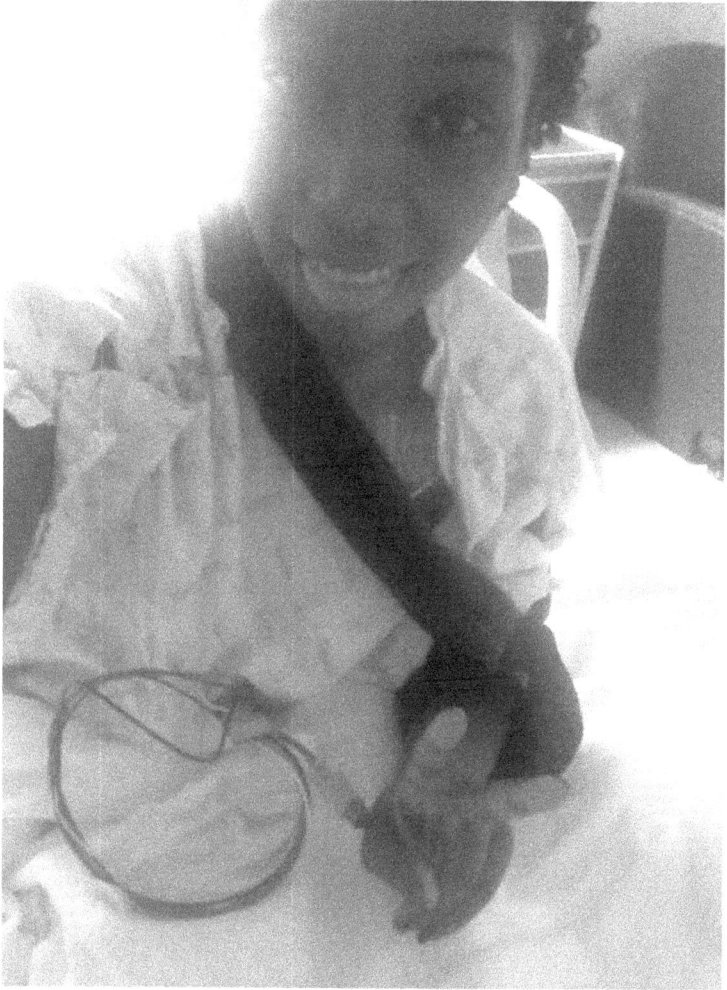

A family photo of my husband and our children.

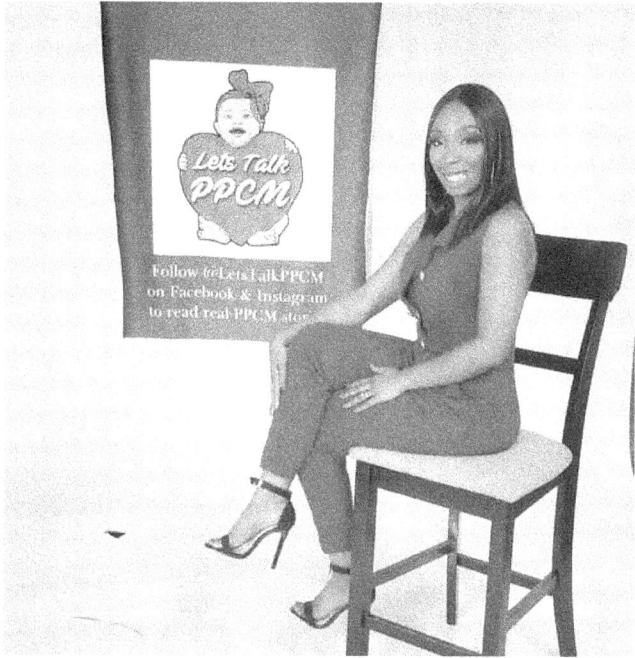

www.ingramcontent.com/pod-product-compliance
Lightning Source LLC
Chambersburg PA
CBHW072201270326
41930CB00011B/2508